Judith L. Fischer, PhD
Miriam Mulsow, PhD
Alan W. Korinek, PhD
Editors

Familial Responses to Alcohol Problems

Familial Responses to Alcohol Problems has been co-published simultaneously as *Alcoholism Treatment Quarterly*, Volume 25, Numbers 1/2 2007.

Pre-publication
REVIEWS,
COMMENTARIES,
EVALUATIONS . . .

"**Q**UALITY ARTICLES emphasizing a relational framework for understanding and treating substance abuse. . . . The life span findings from the Michigan Longitudinal Study are PARTICULARLY VALUABLE for clinicians who see families both before and after substance abuse has been identified. . . . A strong addition to the libraries of experienced therapists and AN EXCELLENT TEACHING TOOL FOR BEGINNING THERAPISTS."

Marcia Lasswell, MS
Past President, American Association of Marriage and Family Therapy
Professor Emeritus
California State University, Pomona

The Haworth Press, Inc.

Familial Responses
to Alcohol Problems

Familial Responses to Alcohol Problems has been co-published simultaneously as *Alcoholism Treatment Quarterly*, Volume 25, Numbers 1/2 2007.

Monographic Separates from *Alcoholism Treatment Quarterly*®

For additional information on these and other Haworth Press titles, including descriptions, tables of contents, reviews, and prices, use the QuickSearch catalog at http://www.HaworthPress.com.

Familial Responses to Alcohol Problems, edited by Judith L. Fischer, PhD, Miriam Mulsow, PhD, and Alan W. Korinek, PhD (Vol. 25, No. 1/2, 2007). *"Quality articles emphasizing a relational framework for understanding and treating substance abuse. . . . The life span findings from the Michigan Longitudinal study are particularly valuable for clinicians who see families both before and after substance abuse has been identified. . . . A strong addition to the libraries of experienced therapists and an excellent teaching tool for beginning therapists." (Marcia Lasswell, MS, Past President, American Association of Marriage and Family Therapy; Professor Emeritus, California State University, Pomona)*

Spirituality and Religiousness and Alcohol/Other Drug Problems: Treatment and Recovery Perspectives, edited by Brent B. Benda, PhD, and Thomas F. McGovern, EdD (Vol. 24, No. 1/2, 2006). *"Convincing evidence that spirituality and religiousness are not only relevant, but integral to our understanding the disease of addiction and the process of recovery." (Dr. Jeffry D. Roth, Editor, Journal of Groups in Addiction and Recovery; Author, Group Psychotherapy and Recovery from Addiction: Carrying the Message)*

Latinos and Alcohol Use/Abuse Revisited: Advances and Challenges for Prevention and Treatment Programs, edited by Melvin Delgado, PhD (Vol. 23, No. 2/3, 2005). *"For anyone interested in building a culturally competent system of care for Latinos, This book will provide invaluable guidance. . . . Fills a substantial gap in our knowledge about alcohol use and abuse among subgroups of Latinos. . . . Brings together research and practice knowledge on a broad range of topics, including the most recent trends in alcohol use and dependence among Latinos, service use and effectiveness, help-seeking behavior and barriers to treatment, the unmet needs of incarcerated Latinos, and ethnically sensitive interventions." (Carol Coohey, PhD, Associate Professor, University of Iowa School of Social Work)*

Responding to Physical and Sexual Abuse in Women with Alcohol and Other Drug and Mental Disorders: Program Building, edited by Bonita M. Veysey, PhD, and Colleen Clark, PhD (Vol. 22, No. 3/4, 2004). *"Highly recommended. Any clinician working with women (and their families) will appreciate the breadth and depth of this book and its use of clinical examples, treatment direction, and sobering statistics." (John Brick, PhD, MA, FAPA, Executive Director, Intoxikon International; Author of Drugs, the Brain, and Behavior and the Handbook of the Medical Consequences of Alcohol and Drug Abuse)*

Alcohol Problems in the United States: Twenty Years of Treatment Perspective, edited by Thomas F. McGovern, EdD, and William L. White, MA (Vol. 20, No. 3/4, 2002). *An overview of trends in the treatment of alcohol problems over a 20-year period.*

Homelessness Prevention in Treatment of Substance Abuse and Mental Illness: Logic Models and Implementation of Eight American Projects, edited by Kendon J. Conrad, PhD, Michael D. Matters, PhD, Patricia Hanrahan, PhD, and Daniel J. Luchins, MD (Vol. 17, No. 1/2, 1999). *Provides you with new insights into how you can help your clients overcome political, economic, and environmental barriers to treatment that can lead to homelessness.*

Alcohol Use/Abuse Among Latinos: Issues and Examples of Culturally Competent Services, edited by Melvin Delgado, PhD (Vol. 16, No. 1/2, 1998). *"This book will have widespread appeal for practitioners and educators involved in direct service delivery, organizational planning, research, or policy development." (Steven Lozano Applewhite, PhD, Associate Professor, Graduate School of Social Work, University of Houston, Texas)*

Treatment of the Addictions: Applications of Outcome Research for Clinical Management, edited by Norman S. Miller, MD (Vol. 12, No. 2, 1994). *"Ambitious and informative . . . Recommended to anybody involved in the practice of substance abuse treatment and research in treatment outcome." (The American Journal of Addictions)*

Self-Recovery: Treating Addictions Using Transcendental Meditation and Maharishi Ayur-Veda, edited by David F. O'Connell, PhD, and Charles N. Alexander, PhD (Vol. 11, No. 1/2/3/4, 1994). *"A scholarly trailblazer, a scientific first. . . . Those who work daily in the fight against substance abuse, violence, and illness will surely profit from reading this important volume. A valuable new tool in what may be America's most difficult battle." (Joseph Drew, PhD, Chair for Evaluation, Mayor's Advisory Committee on Drug Abuse, Washington, DC; Professor of Political Science, University of the District of Columbia)*

Treatment of the Chemically Dependent Homeless: Theory and Implementation in Fourteen American Projects, edited by Kendon J. Conrad, PhD, Cheryl I. Hultman, PhD, and John S. Lyons, PhD (Vol. 10, No. 3/4, 1993). *"A wealth of information and experience. . . . A very useful reference book for everyone seeking to develop their own treatment strategies with this patient group or the homeless mentally ill." (British Journal of Psychiatry)*

Treating Alcoholism and Drug Abuse Among Homeless Men and Women: Nine Community Demonstration Grants, edited by Milton Argeriou, PhD, and Dennis McCarty, PhD (Vol. 7, No. 1, 1990). *"Recommended to those in the process of trying to better serve chemically dependent homeless persons." (Journal of Psychoactive Drugs)*

Co-Dependency: Issues in Treatment and Recovery, edited by Bruce Carruth, PhD, and Warner Mendenhall, PhD (Vol. 6, No. 1, 1989). *"At last a book for clinicians that clearly defines co-dependency and gives helpful treatment approaches. Essential." (Margot Escott, MSW, Social Worker in Private Practice, Naples, Florida)*

The Treatment of Shame and Guilt in Alcoholism Counseling, edited by Ronald T. Potter-Efron, MSW, PhD, and Patricia S. Potter-Efron, MS, CACD III (Vol. 4, No. 2, 1989). *"Comprehensive in its coverage and provides important insights into the treatment of alcoholism, especially the importance to the recovery process of working through feelings of overwhelming shame and guilt. Recommended as required reading." (Australian Psychologist)*

Drunk Driving in America: Strategies and Approaches to Treatment, edited by Stephen K. Valle, ScD, CAC, FACATA (Vol. 3, No. 2, 1986). *Creative and thought-provoking methods related to research, policy, and treatment of the drunk driver.*

Alcohol Interventions: Historical and Sociocultural Approaches, edited by David L. Strug, PhD, S. Priyadarsini, PhD, and Merton M. Hyman (Supp. #1, 1986). *"A comprehensive and unique account of addictions treatment of centuries ago." (Federal Probation: A Journal of Correctional Philosophy)*

Treatment of Black Alcoholics, edited by Frances Larry Brisbane, PhD, MSW, and Maxine Womble, MA (Vol. 2, No. 3/4, 1985). *"Outstanding! In view of the paucity of research on the topic, this text presents some of the outstanding work done in this area." (Dr. Edward R. Smith, Department of Educational Psychology, University of Wisconsin-Milwaukee)*

Psychosocial Issues in the Treatment of Alcoholism, edited by David Cook, CSW, Christine Fewell, ACSW, and Shulamith Lala Ashenberg Straussner, DSW, CEAP (Vol. 2, No. 1, 1985). *"Well-written and informative; the topic areas are relevant to today's social issues and offer some new approaches to the treatment of alcoholics." (The American Journal of Occupational Therapy)*

Alcoholism and Sexual Dysfunction: Issues in Clinical Management, edited by David J. Powell, PhD (Vol. 1, No. 3, 1984). *"It does a good job of explicating the linkage between two of the most common health problems in the U.S. today." (Journal of Sex & Marital Therapy)*

Familial Responses to Alcohol Problems

Judith L. Fischer, PhD
Miriam Mulsow, PhD
Alan W. Korinek, PhD
Editors

Familial Responses to Alcohol Problems has been co-published simultaneously as *Alcoholism Treatment Quarterly*, Volume 25, Numbers 1/2 2007.

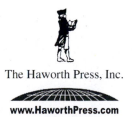

The Haworth Press, Inc.
www.HaworthPress.com

Familial Responses to Alcohol Problems has been co-published simultaneously as *Alcoholism Treatment Quarterly*, Volume 25, Numbers 1/2 2007.

The development, preparation, and publication of this work has been undertaken with great care. However, the publisher, employees, editors, and agents of The Haworth Press and all imprints of The Haworth Press, Inc., including The Haworth Medical Press® and Pharmaceutical Products Press®, are not responsible for any errors contained herein or for consequences that may ensue from use of materials or information contained in this work. With regard to case studies, identities and circumstances of individuals discussed herein have been changed to protect confidentiality. Any resemblance to actual persons, living or dead, is entirely coincidental.

The Haworth Press is committed to the dissemination of ideas and information according to the highest standards of intellectual freedom and the free exchange of ideas. Statements made and opinions expressed in this publication do not necessarily reflect the views of the Publisher, Directors, management, or staff of The Haworth Press, Inc., or an endorsement by them.

The Haworth Press, Inc., 10 Alice Street, Binghamton, 13904-1580 USA

Cover design by Jennifer M. Gaska

Library of Congress Cataloging-in-Publication Data

Familial responses to alcohol problems / Judith L. Fischer, Miriam Mulsow, Alan W. Korinek, editors.
     p. cm.
     "Familial Responses to Alcohol Problems has been co-published simultaneously as Alcoholism Treatment Quarterly, Volume 25, Numbers 1/2 2007."
     Includes bibliographical references and index.
     ISBN-13: 978-0-7890-3515-8 (hard cover : alk. paper)
     ISBN-10: 0-7890-3515-4 (hard cover : alk. paper)
     ISBN-13: 978-0-7890-3516-5 (soft cover : alk. paper)
     ISBN-10: 0-7890-3516-2 (soft cover : alk. paper)
     1. Alcoholics–Family relationships–United States. 2. Alcoholism–Treatment–United States. I. Fischer, Judith L. II. Mulsow, Miriam. III. Korinek, Alan W. IV. Alcoholism treatment quarterly.
     HV5132.F344 2007
     362.29'23–dc22
                                                  2006030008

The HAWORTH PRESS Inc.
Abstracting, Indexing & Outward Linking
PRINT and ELECTRONIC BOOKS & JOURNALS

This section provides you with a list of major indexing & abstracting services and other tools for bibliographic access. That is to say, each service began covering this periodical during the year noted in the right column. Most Websites which are listed below have indicated that they will either post, disseminate, compile, archive, cite or alert their own Website users with research-based content from this work. (This list is as current as the copyright date of this publication.)

Abstracting, Website/Indexing Coverage . . . . Year When Coverage Began

- **Academic Search Premier (EBSCO)**
  <http://search.ebscohost.com> 1995
- **CINAHL (Cumulative Index to Nursing & Allied Health
  Literature) (EBSCO)** <http://www.cinahl.com> 2007
- **EMBASE Excerpta Medica (Elsevier)**
  <http://www.elsevier.nl> 1984
- **EMBASE.com (The Power of EMBASE + MEDLINE Combined)
  (Elsevier)** <http://www.embase.com> . . . . *
- **MasterFILE Premier (EBSCO)**
  <http://search.ebscohost.com> 1995
- **Psychological Abstracts (PsycINFO)** <http://www.apa.org> . . . 1984
- **Social Services Abstracts (ProQuest CSA)**
  <http://www.csa.com> 1990
- **Social Work Abstracts (NASW)**
  <http://www.silverplatter.com/catalog/swab.htm> 1991
- **Sociological Abstracts (ProQuest CSA)**
  <http://www.csa.com> 1990
- Abstracts in Anthropology <http://www.baywood.com/
  Journals/PreviewJournals.asp?Id=0001-3455> 1991
- Academic Search Alumni Edition (EBSCO)
  <http://search.ebscohost.com> 2007

(continued)

(continued)

(continued)

Bibliographic Access

- *ATForum.com <http://www.atforum.com>*

- *Cabell's Directory of Publishing Opportunities in Psychology <http://www.cabells.com>*

- *MediaFinder <http://www.mediafinder.com/>*

- *Ulrich's Periodicals Directory: The Global Source for Periodicals Information Since 1932 <http://www.bowkerlink.com>*

Special Bibliographic Notes related to special journal issues (separates) and indexing/abstracting:

- indexing/abstracting services in this list will also cover material in any "separate" that is co-published simultaneously with Haworth's special thematic journal issue or DocuSerial. Indexing/abstracting usually covers material at the article/chapter level.
- monographic co-editions are intended for either non-subscribers or libraries which intend to purchase a second copy for their circulating collections.
- monographic co-editions are reported to all jobbers/wholesalers/approval plans. The source journal is listed as the "series" to assist the prevention of duplicate purchasing in the same manner utilized for books-in-series.
- to facilitate user/access services all indexing/abstracting services are encouraged to utilize the co-indexing entry note indicated at the bottom of the first page of each article/chapter/contribution.
- this is intended to assist a library user of any reference tool (whether print, electronic, online, or CD-ROM) to locate the monographic version if the library has purchased this version but not a subscription to the source journal.
- individual articles/chapters in any Haworth publication are also available through the Haworth Document Delivery Service (HDDS).

As part of Haworth's continuing commitment to better serve our library patrons, we are proud to be working with the following electronic services:

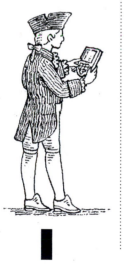

AGGREGATOR SERVICES

EBSCOhost

Ingenta

J-Gate

Minerva

OCLC FirstSearch

Oxmill

SwetsWise

LINK RESOLVER SERVICES

1Cate (Openly Informatics)

ChemPort
(American Chemical Society)

CrossRef

Gold Rush (Coalliance)

LinkOut (PubMed)

LINKplus (Atypon)

LinkSolver (Ovid)

LinkSource with A-to-Z (EBSCO)

Resource Linker (Ulrich)

SerialsSolutions (ProQuest)

SFX (Ex Libris)

Sirsi Resolver (SirsiDynix)

Tour (TDnet)

Vlink (Extensity, formerly Geac)

WebBridge (Innovative Interfaces)

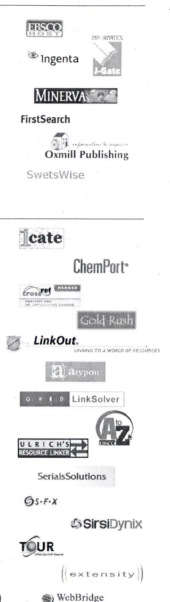

Familial Responses
to Alcohol Problems

CONTENTS

ABOUT THE EDITORS

Judith L. Fischer, PhD, is Professor of Human Development and Family Studies at Texas Tech University, Lubbock, Texas. She was honored as the first C.W. and Virginia Hutcheson Professor in Human Development and Family Studies, 2001-2003. She received the Texas Tech President's Academic Achievement Award in 1998, and is a three time awardee of the College of Human Sciences Researcher of the Year award. She served as department chair, 1993-1999, and as President of the Groves Conference on Marriage and Family, 1996-1999. Her research concerns family problems and problems of adolescents and young adults with substance use and misuse. Currently, she serves on the Editorial Boards of *Journal of Marriage and Family*, *Personal Relationships*, *Journal of Social and Personal Relationships*, and *Journal of Early Adolescence*, and as occasional reviewer for *Journal of Studies on Alcohol*. Her research has been supported by NICHD research grants. She has published more than 60 articles and chapters in a wide range of family, addictions, and interpersonal relationships journals and books.

Miriam Mulsow, PhD, is Director of Graduate Programs and Associate Professor of Human Development and Family Studies at Texas Tech University, Lubbock, Texas. She was awarded a Fulbright-Hays Group Study Abroad Fellowship for study in Cambodia, Laos, and Vietnam during Summer, 2004. She served on the Board of Directors 1999-2002 and 2004-2008 and as 2006 Program Vice President of the Texas Council on Family Relations and was selected for the National Council on Family Relations Association of Councils Meritorious Service Award in 2001. Her research concerns family stress, parenting stress, and trauma including dealing with ADHD, substance abuse, maltreatment, and PTSD in families. She has served as a reviewer for *Journal of Marital and Family Therapy* and *Journal of Family Issues*, and as a grant reviewer for the Canadian Mental Health Association. She also served on the Hogg Foundation Evaluation Initiative.

Alan W. Korinek, PhD, is Director of the Employee Assistance Program, Southwest Institute for Addictive Diseases, Department of Neuropsychiatry, Texas Tech University Health Sciences Center, Lubbock, Texas. His research concerns include organizational interventions, dynamics of intimate relationships, and spirituality. He has published several articles on these and other topics.

Family Systems, Biopsychosocial Processes, and Lifespan Development: Introduction to Family Response to Alcohol Problems

Judith L. Fischer, PhD
Alan Korinek, PhD
Miriam Mulsow, PhD

SUMMARY. This volume reviews literature, research programs, and therapy approaches to family response to alcohol. Three articles view the topic from particular points in the lifespan: childhood (Fitzgerald, Puttler, Refior, & Zucker), adolescence and youth (Fischer, Pidcock, & Fletcher-Stephens), and older age (Stelle & Scott). Five articles cover specific topics on families, highlighting (a) processes to involve an

---

Judith L. Fischer is affiliated with the Dept. of Human Development and Family Studies, Texas Tech University, Box 41162, Lubbock, TX 79409-1162 (E-mail: judith.fischer@ttu.edu).

Alan Korinek is Director of the Employee Assistance Program, Southwest Institute of Addictive Diseases, Dept. of Neuropsychiatry, Texas Tech University Health Sciences Center, Lubbock, TX (E-mail: alan.korinek@ttuhsc.edu).

Miriam Mulsow is Associate Professor and Graduate Program Director, Dept. of Human Development and Family Studies, Texas Tech University, Box 41162, Lubbock, TX 79409-1162 (E-mail: miriam.mulsow@ttu.edu).

Address correspondence to: Judith L. Fischer at the above address.

[Haworth co-indexing entry note]: "Family Systems, Biopsychosocial Processes, and Lifespan Development: Introduction to Family Response to Alcohol Problems." Fischer, Judith L., Alan Korinek, and Miriam Mulsow. Co-published simultaneously in *Alcoholism Treatment Quarterly* (The Haworth Press, Inc.) Vol. 25, No. 1/2, 2007, pp. 1-9; and: *Familial Responses to Alcohol Problems* (ed: Judith L. Fischer, Miriam Mulsow, and Alan W. Korinek) The Haworth Press, Inc., 2007, pp. 1-9. Single or multiple copies of this article are available for a fee from The Haworth Document Delivery Service [1-800-HAWORTH, 9:00 a.m. - 5:00 p.m. (EST). E-mail address: docdelivery@haworthpress.com].

Available online at http://atq.haworthpress.com
doi:10.1300/J020v25n01_01

1

alcoholic family member in treatment (Garrett & Landau), (b) couples (Navarra), (c) families with children (Lewis & Allen-Byrd), (d) co-morbidity in families (Mulsow), and (e) spirituality as a family endeavor (Korinek). doi:10.1300/J020v25n01_01 *[Article copies available for a fee from The Haworth Document Delivery Service: 1-800-HAWORTH. E-mail address: <docdelivery@haworthpress.com> Website: <http://www.HaworthPress.com> © 2007 by The Haworth Press, Inc. All rights reserved.]*

KEYWORDS. Family systems, biopsychosocial, alcohol, lifespan

INTRODUCTION

In their journal *Family Dynamics of Addiction Quarterly*, Lawson and Lawson (1991) described the history of the emerging field of addictions and family systems thus: "In only three decades the field has evolved from the belief that alcoholism is a moral weakness, or, at best, an individual pathology to an understanding that addictions are many, complex, and best understood from a systems perspective, especially an intergenerational systems perspective" (p. 59). The earliest cited articles in their annotated review of classic studies in the field of family dynamics of addiction focused on the wives of alcoholic men (cf., Jackson, 1954; Whalen, 1953). By the late 1960's and early 1970's, research included additional family members, such as parents and siblings (cf., Klimenko, 1968; Schuckit, Goodwin, & Winokur, 1972; Smart & Fejer, 1972). Involved in integrating the fields of alcoholism and family systems were such early pioneers as Bateson (1971), Bowen (1974), Jacob (Jacob, Favorini, Meisel, & Anderson, 1978), Moos (Moos, Bromet, Tsu, & Moos, 1979; Moos & Moos, 1976), and Steinglass (Steinglass, 1976, 1980; Steinglass & Wolin, 1974; Steinglass, Weiner, & Mendelson, 1979). In 1987, the influential book *The Alcoholic Family* was published (Steinglass, Bennett, Wolin, & Reiss 1987). About this time, the National Institute on Alcohol Abuse and Alcoholism (NIAAA) brought together prominent researchers in the field to produce the edited volume *The Development of Alcohol Problems: Exploring the Biopsychosocial Matrix of Risk* (Zucker, Boyd, & Howard, 1994). The chapters in this book focused attention on the interplay of biology and genetics, psychological processes, and social influences, including families, on the development of alcohol problems.

This volume draws upon the perspectives from family systems theory and from the biopsychosocial model in its choice of topics and in its organizing framework. The lifespan ranges from prenatal to late old age. At each time in the lifespan, biopsychosocial processes are engaged. Biological and genetic processes include inherited propensities, physiological responses to alcohol, and temperament. Psychological processes involve personality, attitudes, expectations, emotion regulation, and social skills. Social influences include interpersonal relationships with other people, as well as embeddedness within social settings. Other people are often parents, siblings, children, peers, romantic partners, and those with specific roles such as teachers, mentors, colleagues, and even enemies. Social settings include family, neighborhood, support networks, and settings for spiritual development and recovery, as well as institutions involving places of education, work, worship, governing, and healing.

The primary focus in this collection is on family response to alcohol (see Garrett & Landau, this volume, for a definition of family). Topics highlighting family involvement were selected to describe situations when (a) parents have the disease of alcoholism that impacts their children and other relatives, (b) parents interact with children to prevent or to reduce a child's involvement with alcohol, (c) there are attempts to involve a family member in seeking help with alcoholism, (d) children recognize and intervene in a parent's alcohol misuse, (e) couples enter into recovery and deal with issues involving each other and their children, (f) the co-occurrence of other disorders disrupts family life, and (g) recovery includes attention to spiritual development.

Of necessity, choices had to made as to what to include and what to exclude in this volume. Early plans called for an article on codependency. Although these issues could be, and were, subsumed in more general discussions of couple and family dynamics, a stand alone article on codependency as a family response to alcohol would have continued a tradition of publishing works in this journal that advance the field. Interested readers are directed to such sources as Crothers and Warren (1994), Fischer and Crawford, (1992), Fischer, Spann, and Crawford (1991), Fischer, Wampler, Lyness, and Thomas (1991), and Wright and Wright (1990, 1999).

Likewise, though our desire was to cover the lifespan, the topic of prenatal exposure to alcohol and resulting fetal alcohol effects (FAE) and fetal alcohol syndrome (FAS) infants, was not included. Although some symptoms and problems may differ between FAS, FAE, and "crack" babies, the general portrait is one of developmental deficits in learning, motor skills, and social skills, as well as attention deficits and hyperactivity (Thomas & Riley, 1998). Already vulnerable infants may be growing up in families impacted in other ways by parental alcoholism. Treatment for pregnant substance-abusing women suffers from underfunding, lack of facilities in general, and lack of facilities that accept Medicaid or have child care (McMurtrie, Rosenberg, Kerker, Kan, & Graham, 1999).

Other excluded topics that involve families and alcoholism, such as diversity and alcoholism (Delgado, 2005; McGovern & White, 2002) and physical and sexual abuse in women (Veysey & Clark, 2004), have received attention from this journal in very recent issues; thus, we did not ask authors to revisit them specifically in the present articles. Other topics, such as biological and genetic factors, are not given a single focus, but are referenced or inferred in many of the current articles.

Despite space restrictions that limited the scope of this volume, we believe we have recruited articles from scholars that highlight some of the most exciting work in the field today. The article by Fitzgerald, Puttler, Refior, and Zucker describes a long-term research project, the Michigan Longitudinal Study, that has traced the lives of community children with alcoholic and nonalcoholic parents from very young ages (3-5 years) through current adolescence. Importantly, this project is based on a risk-cumulating model that demonstrates how a theory driven project can pay big dividends in illuminating the processes by which young children with alcoholic parents traverse the challenges of childhood and adolescence. It brings home how important it is to have a fuller understanding of the kind of alcoholism the parent displays (anti-social and non-anti-social) since that has a profound effect on the developmental course of these offspring. The article also provides insight into three developmental pathways of children, one characterized by considerable continuity and two others that reflect divergence of development in middle childhood.

Adolescence and youth can be treacherous times when alcohol, family and outside influences mix. Fischer, Pidcock, and Fletcher-Stephens provide an overview of the alcohol-specific and non-alcohol-specific family issues with respect to adolescent alcohol use and misuse. The authors note the influence, and limits on influence, of parental substance use and abuse on adolescent alcohol misuse. In addition, three important researched-based approaches to treating adolescent alcohol use problems in a family context are reviewed: Multisystemic Therapy, Brief Strategic Therapy, and Multidimensional Family Therapy.

A number of people in adolescence and adulthood encounter periods of heavy involvement with alcohol with troubling consequences for themselves and those involved with them. However, for some people the problems associated with alcohol abuse are also experienced, or first experienced, in the later years of life. Using family systems theory, Stelle and Scott provide an overview that describes the "invisible epidemic" of alcohol abuse by older family members. The authors detail the issues involved in screening, detection, and diagnosis in this population. Family level interventions are described and evaluated. As these authors note, "a family involved approach is not necessarily a systems focus...."

The next three articles center more extensively on treatment issues for (primarily) adults who abuse alcohol: how to bring the family member into treatment (Garrett & Landau); what couples have to say about their experiences with alcoholism in a spouse (Navarra); and what families and family members, including children, encounter as they go through the course of family recovery (Lewis & Allen-Byrd). As these three articles illustrate, the whole family is involved in the process of recovery, not just the recovering individual. Garrett and Landau address their concept of Family Motivation to Change in their ARISE method to "get a resistant individual with a drinking problem started in treatment." They provide a research substantiated approach to helping the person they term the First Caller to bring the person with the alcohol problem into contact with professionals. Their case example extends beyond the United States to a war-torn part of Europe, Kosova.

Navarra's article shares the results of research on his Couples Reciprocal Development Approach (CRDA) with couples in long term recovery. In their focus group meetings, Navarra's couples share insights and struggles as they engage the process of recovery. Evolving issues are identified as residing in three core areas: couple identity, family of origin issues, and couple interdependence. Lewis and Allen-Byrd identify and describe the three stages that families encounter as they advance in recovery from Transition to Early Recovery to Ongoing Recovery. In each stage, therapist approaches to the family in recovery are illustrated. In this paper, coping strategies presented by the therapist are outlined and emerging issues in family therapy and recovery are identified. As their article illustrates, it is not just the spouse of an alcoholic who has recovery issues to deal with, but the children in the family as well.

Comorbidity can be a tricky issue, not just in the development of alcohol problems, but in diagnosis and treatment. Mulsow provides a review of these issues focusing particularly on four common comorbid diagnoses with alcohol problems: ADHD, trauma, anxiety disorders, and mood disorders. She reviews family issues involved in the treatment of comorbid conditions.

As the articles in this collection illustrate, family members have important roles to play in alcohol misuse maintenance and recovery. One of the ways in which family members can be involved in recovery is through family spirituality (Korinek). Individual spirituality has long been a feature of such recovery programs as Alcoholics Anonymous. Family spirituality engages the whole family in spiritual growth and development. Korinek describes family meditation, prayer, restoration of rituals, confession and forgiveness, service to others, and religious involvement as possible avenues for family spiritual development. In addition, he provides a case example and a nuanced description of how and when spiritual issues may be undertaken in family recovery.

The authors of the articles in this volume bring a wide range of experiences and expertise. Some are written by researcher/therapists who are actively engaged in helping clients deal with recovery in a family context and/or in helping to train others to provide these important functions (Garrett & Landau; Korinek; Lewis; Navarra; Pidcock & Fletcher-Stephens). Others provide descriptions of research and research programs that have important implications for prevention and treatment (Fitzgerald et al., Fischer et al., Mulsow, Stelle & Scott).

There are a number of controversies and challenges in the field of families and alcoholism. Some of these challenges are: the need for more research to support evidence-based practice; whether disease mechanisms are at work in the nonalcoholic family member; what are appropriate prescription and physician administered drugs for a recovering alcoholic with a comorbid diagnosis or with a health emergency that requires anesthesia and pain management; provisions for child welfare and family reunification if children are removed from the home; issues of causation, for example, refraining from blaming the victim, whether that is the actively drinking person in the family or other family members; and the role of genetics. If a gene (or combination of gene mechanisms) for alcoholism is found, what are the implications for prevention and treatment and for family planning decisions? Even such basics as terminology can meet with controversy. We understand that some would prefer the descriptor 'person with alcoholism' to 'alcoholic'; in this volume both terms were used by the authors of the articles.

As we worked on this publication we are mindful of the severe problems facing families in the areas of prevention and therapy. There are not enough funds, not enough treatment centers, and not enough understanding of the problems of alcoholism and alcohol misuse. Although the professional field may have evolved from an emphasis on individual morality and pathology to a systems understanding of alcohol problems, the political landscape seems hostile to using the results of science to help the family members who struggle with addiction. Although family-based approaches have been advocated (Edwards & Steinglass, 1995; Samford, Vaughn, Shumway, Jefferies, & Arredondo, 2001; Steinglass, Tislenko, & Reiss, 1985), many insurance companies are still reluctant to reimburse clinicians and programs using these approaches. They prefer instead to recognize only individual-based treatments for alcoholism.

The articles in these pages provide state of the art endeavors. Nonetheless, we understand that this volume is only a start in what promises to be a long term engagement between families and alcohol. In closing, we thank Thomas McGovern, *Alcoholism Treatment Quarterly* editor, for entrusting us with this volume.

REFERENCES

Bateson, G. (1971). The cybernetics of "self ": A theory of alcoholism. *Psychiatry, 34,* 1-18.*

Bowen, M. (1974). Alcoholism as viewed through family systems theory and family psychotherapy. *Annals of the New York Academy of Sciences, 233,* 115-122.*

Crothers, M., & Warren, L. W. (1994). Parental antecedents of adult codependency. *Journal of Clinical Psychology, 52*(2), 231-239.

Delgado, M. (Ed.). (2005). Latinos and alcohol use/abuse revisited: Advances and challenges for prevention and treatment programs. *Alcoholism Treatment Quarterly, 23*(2/3).

Edwards, M. E., & Steinglass, P. (1995). Family therapy treatment outcomes for alcoholism. *Journal of Marital and Family Therapy, 21,* 475-509.

Fischer, J. L., & Crawford, D. (1992). Codependency and parenting styles. *Journal of Adolescent Research, 7,* 352-363.

Fischer, J. L., Spann, L., & Crawford, D. (1991). Measuring codependency. *Alcoholism Treatment Quarterly, 8,* 87-100.

Fischer, J. L., Wampler, R., Lyness, K., & Thomas, E. M. (1992). Offspring codependency: Blocking the impact of family of origin. *Family Dynamics of Addiction Quarterly, 2,* 20-32.

Jackson, J. K. (1954). The adjustment of the family to the crisis of alcoholism. *Quarterly Journal of Studies on Alcohol, 15,* 562-586.*

Jacob, T., Favorini, A., Meisel, S. S., & Anderson, C. M. (1978). The alcoholic's spouse, children and family interactions: Substantive findings and methodological issues. *Journal of Studies on Alcohol, 39,* 1231-1251.*

Klimenko, A. (1968). Multifamily therapy in the rehabilitation of drug addicts. *Perspective on Psychiatric Care, 6*, 220-223.*

Lawson, A. W., & Lawson, G. W. (1991). Classic articles in the field of family dynamics of addiction: The early years, 1953-1980. *Family Dynamics of Addiction Quarterly, 1*, 59-70.

McGovern, T. F., & White, W. L. (Eds.). (2002). Alcohol problems in the United States: Twenty years of treatment perspective. *Alcoholism Treatment Quarterly, 20*(3/4).

McMurtrie, C., Rosenberg, K. D., Kerker, B. D., Kan, J., & Graham, E. H. (1999). A unique drug treatment program for pregnant and postpartum substance-using women in New York City: Results of a pilot project, 1990-1995. *American Journal of Drug and Alcohol Abuse, 25*, 701-713.

Moos, R. H., Bromet, E., Tsu, V., & Moos, B. (1979). Family characteristics and the outcome of treatment for alcoholism. *Journal of Studies on Alcohol, 40*, 78-88.*

Moos, R. H., & Moos, B. S. (1976). A typology of family social environments. *Family Process, 15*, 357-371.*

Samford, B., Vaughn, M., Shumway, S., Jefferies, V., & Arredondo, R. (2001). Treating individuals and families for alcohol/other drug problems in an intensive outpatient setting. *Alcoholism Treatment Quarterly, 19*, 65-80.

Shuckit, M. A., Goodwin, D. A., & Winokur, G. (1972). A study of alcoholism in half siblings. *American Journal of Psychiatry, 128*, 1132-1136.*

Smart, R., & Fejer, D. (1972). Drug use among adolescents and their parents: Closing the generation gap in mood modification. *Journal of Abnormal Psychology, 79*, 153-160.*

Steinglass, P. (1976). Experimenting with family treatment approaches to alcoholism, 1950-1975: A review. *Family Process, 15*, 97-123.*

Steinglass, P. (1980). A life history model of the alcoholic family. *Family Process, 19*, 211-225.*

Steinglass, P., Bennett, L. A., Wolin, S. J., & Reiss, D. (1987). *The alcoholic family.* New York: BasicBooks.

Steinglass, P., Davis, D. I., & Berenson, D. (1977). Observations of conjointly hospitalized alcoholic couples during sobriety and intoxication: Implications for theory and therapy. *Family Process, 16*, 1-16.*

Steinglass, P., Tislenko, L., & Reiss, D. (1985). Stability/instability in the alcoholic marriage: The interrelationships between course of alcoholism, family process, and marital outcome. *Family Process, 24*, 365-376.

Steinglass, P., Weiner, S., & Mendelson, J. A. (1979). A systems approach to alcoholism: A model and its clinical application. *Archives of General Psychiatry, 24*, 401-408.*

Steinglass, P., & Wolin, S. (1974). Explorations of a systems approach to alcoholism. *Archives of General Psychiatry, 31*, 527-532.*

Thomas, J. D., & Riley, E. P. (1998). Fetal alcohol syndrome. *Alcohol Health & Research World, 22*, 47-54.

Veysey, B. M., & Clark, C. (Eds.). (2004). Responding to physical and sexual abuse in women with alcohol and other drug and mental disorders: Program building. *Alcoholism Treatment Quarterly, 22*(3/4).

Whalen, T. (1953). Wives of alcoholics: Four types observed in a family service agency. *Quarterly Journal of Studies on Alcohol, 14*, 632-641.*

Wright, P. H. & Wright, K. D. (1990). Measuring codependents' close relationships: A preliminary study. *Journal of Substance Abuse, 2*, 335-344.

Wright, P. H. & Wright, K. D. (1999). The two faces of codependent relating: A research-based perspective. *Contemporary Family Therapy, 21*, 527-542.

Zucker, R., Boyd, G., & Howard, J. (1994). *The development of alcohol problems: Exploring the biopsychosocial matrix of risk* (National Institute on Alcohol Abuse and Alcoholism Research Monograph No. 26). Rockville, MD: U. S. Department of Health and Human Services.

* denotes articles annotated in Lawson & Lawson, 1991.

doi:10.1300/J020v25n01_01

Family Response to Children and Alcohol

Hiram E. Fitzgerald, PhD
Leon I. Puttler, PhD
Susan Refior, MSW
Robert A. Zucker, PhD

SUMMARY. We describe the Michigan Longitudinal Study (MLS), an etiologic study of family risk for alcoholism over the life course, and provide an overview of findings from the first 12 years of the study. Data suggest that etiology is anchored in family diathesis and shaped by a wide range of experiences that structure differential developmental pathways. One pathway is marked by strong continuity of behavioral dysregulation, evident during the preschool years and continuing through early adolescence. Two discontinuous pathways illustrate the shifting nature of risk

Hiram E. Fitzgerald is affiliated with the Department of Psychology and University Outreach and Engagement, Kellogg Center, Garden Level, Michigan State University, East Lansing, MI 48824 (E-mail: fitzger9@msu.edu).

Leon I. Puttler and Susan Refior are affiliated with the Department of Psychiatry and the Addiction Research Center, University of Michigan (E-mail: puttler@msu.edu; refior@msu.edu).

Robert A. Zucker is affiliated with the Departments of Psychiatry, Psychology and the Addiction Research Center, University of Michigan, 2025 Traverwood Drive Suite A, Ann Arbor, MI 48105-7995 (E-mail: zuckerra@umich.edu).

Work reported in this article was supported by NIAAA Grants R37 AA07065 to RAZ & HEF R01 AA12217 to RAZ & JTN.

Address correspondence to: Hiram E. Fitzgerald, PhD, University Outreach and Engagement, Kellogg Center Garden Level, Michigan State University, East Lansing, MI 48824 (E-mail: fitzger9@msu.edu).

[Haworth co-indexing entry note]: "Family Response to Children and Alcohol." Fitzgerald, Hiram E. et al. Co-published simultaneously in *Alcoholism Treatment Quarterly* (The Haworth Press, Inc.) Vol. 25, No. 1/2, 2007, pp. 11-25; and: *Familial Responses to Alcohol Problems* (ed: Judith L. Fischer, Miriam Mulsow, and Alan W. Korinek) The Haworth Press, Inc., 2007, pp. 11-25. Single or multiple copies of this article are available for a fee from The Haworth Document Delivery Service [1-800-HAWORTH, 9:00 a.m. - 5:00 p.m. (EST). E-mail address: docdelivery@haworthpress.com].

and protective factors during early human development. Paternal co-morbid psychopathology, antisocial behavior, and alcoholism, play critical roles not only with respect to parent-child relationships, but also as determinants of family functioning and family stability. Implications for linking prevention efforts to developmental pathways are suggested. doi:10.1300/

J020v25n01_02 [Article copies available for a fee from The Haworth Document Delivery Service: 1-800-HAWORTH. E-mail address: <docdelivery@haworthpress. com> Website: <http://www.HaworthPress.com> © 2007 by The Haworth Press, Inc. All rights reserved.]

KEYWORDS. Alcoholism, early onset, risk cumulation, resilience, emergent pathways

INTRODUCTION

Approximately 20 million American adults are alcoholic and many of them are parents of an estimated 28 million children, 2,340,000 of whom are between the ages of birth and six years old (SAMHSA, 1998). Children of alcoholics (COAs) are at least 6 times greater risk for alcohol abuse than are children with no family history of alcoholism (Grant, 2000). By age 14, half of the children in the United States report that they had their first drink, excluding drinks associated with religious or family celebrations. Adolescents who use alcohol at earlier ages are 4 times more likely to become alcohol dependent than are individuals who delay use to about age 20 (Grant & Dawson, 1997). While prevalence rates are increasing, the time between first use and onset of problem drinking is becoming shorter (Tarter & Vanyukov, 1994). Exposure to family alcoholism increases children's risk for the development of an alcohol use disorder, and as we will illustrate in this article, exposure to an alcoholic family environment also exacerbates risk for co-occurring psychopathology.

THE MICHIGAN LONGITUDINAL STUDY (MLS)

The MLS has been following community-recruited families for nearly two decades in a prospective study that is focused on the identification of risk and protective factors related to alcoholism over the life course (Zucker & Fitzgerald, 1991). Families were originally recruited into the study from four counties in mid-Michigan. This population based sampling of non-Hispanic Caucasian families consisted of high risk (court recruited), moderate risk (community recruited alcoholics) and low risk families (nonalcoholics). (See Fitzgerald, Zucker & Yang, 1995; Zucker, Fitzgerald & Moses, 1995; Zucker et al., 2000, for additional details about study recruitment.)

Data are collected every three years beginning when the children are between 3 and 5 years of age. When children reach 11 years of age, brief annual assessments also take place and continue through age 17. Although both boys and girls are included in the sample, recruitment of girls did not occur in synchrony with that of boys. Thus, sample size for determining effects on daughters of alcoholics is not yet sufficient for the complex analyses required for demonstrating longitudinal effects. Therefore, in this article we focus on results from the MLS that are specific to sons.

Comparisons among the three recruitment groups indicated that alcoholic families were functioning at poorer levels at the beginning of the study. For example, court recruited alcoholic families had lower family income, lower occupational prestige indicators of socio-economic status, and less paternal and maternal education than comparison families. Fathers were more depressed, were involved with more antisocial behavior, had higher lifetime alcohol use, and poorer general functioning than community controls (Zucker et al., 2000). Moreover, social visibility of alcoholism was positively correlated with census tract prevalence rates of poverty, divorce/separation, female head of household, family receipt of public assistance, unemployment, and renter occupied households (Zucker et al., 2000). We refer to this embeddedness of individual, in family, and in community as reflecting the "restedness" of factors that must be considered in any developmental or etiologic models of alcoholism. Assuming some degree of genetic risk, all of the subsequent experiential factors become nested within the matrix of influences that serve to structure diverse developmental pathways.

Very early in the study, we moved from the original recruitment groupings to groupings that reflected person-environment relationships based on the presence or absence of fathers' lifetime antisociality as a differentiating characteristic among the alcoholic families (Zucker, Ellis & Fitzgerald, 1994). Our decision was based on the high comorbidity of alcoholism with other psychiatric problems, particularly antisocial personality disorder for men. Alcoholism with comorbid antisocial behavior is related to earlier onset of alcoholic disorder, with higher levels of other psychopathology, and with a denser family history of alcoholism in the pedigree (Babor, 1996; Zucker, Ellis, Bingham, Fitzgerald & Sanford, 1996). The power of this differentiating factor led us to formulate three groups, and the exploration of the ways that this grouping variable affects history, course, and outcomes for the children as well as the parents has been one of the major foci of the study to date. The family groups, defined solely by father characteristics, are antisocial alcoholics (AALs), non-antisocial alcoholics (NAALs), and Controls. Maternal characteristics are important in analyses related to child outcomes, but they were not the basis for either initial recruitment or family-group formation, although later analyses showed strong relationships between marital psychopathology and the father based groupings (Ichiyama, Zucker, Fitzgerald, & Bingham, 1996; Jester, Zucker, Wong, & Fitzgerald, 2000). Because alcoholism diagnosis can vary from one longitudinal wave to another (cf. McAweeney et al., 2005), the sample size for AALs and NAALs varies depending on the alcoholism diagnosis, but AALs have always comprised the smaller alcoholic group and are most likely to have been court recruited.

The MLS was designed to identify pathways to alcoholism (Zucker & Fitzgerald 1991), to specify the determinants of those pathways (Zucker et al., 1995), and to generate recommendations for policy and prevention based on scientific knowledge of etiology (Zucker, et al., 2000; Zucker & Wong, 2004). To date, findings from the MSL indicate that there are multiple pathways leading to alcoholism and co-active psychopathology, and that these pathways are identifiable during the early years of childhood (Zucker et al., 1995), and most probably have origins that are anchored in genetic and congenital risk (Carmichael-Olson, O'Connor, & Fitzgerald, 1999; Fuller et al., 2003; Zucker, in press).

CONCEPTUAL FRAMEWORK

The conceptual framework guiding the MLS is a risk-cumulation model. It posits that as aggressive behavior, negative emotions, and alcohol involvement accumulate and become ierconnected, children become increasingly at risk for substance abuse disorders, particularly, alcohol use disorders (Zucker, 1987; Zucker, Chermack & Curran, 2000). We conceptualize etiology from a probabilistic biopsychosocial or systems approach (Fitzgerald, Davies, Zucker, & Klinger, 1994; Fitzgerald, et al., 1995; Zucker, 1987, 1989, in press), which emphasizes identification of unique pathways of development and variation in life course that exacerbate risk or provide protection against it. From this risk cumulative perspective, risk for alcoholism is organized within the inter-dynamics of individual, familial and social environment variables. Because contextual events play a critical role in the organization, disorganization, and reorganization of developmental pathways, neither resilience nor risk can be viewed as fixed attributes of the individual (Zucker, Wong, Puttler & Fitzgerald, 2003). Thus, the challenge is to identify variables that maintain or canalize developmental pathways; those that shift individuals from one pathway to another over the course of development and those that predict the life course at various time periods over the life span.

CHARACTERISTICS OF THE PARENTAL REARING ENVIRONMENT

Antisocial alcoholic families provide a rearing environment that creates a high level of risk, including a history of parental regulatory dysfunction and psychopathology (Fitzgerald et al., 2002). For example, the parents of AAL families are more likely to have a history of childhood behavior problems, illegal behavior, frequent arrests, chronic lying, relationship disturbances, depression, neuroticism, poor achievement and cognitive functioning, and low socioecononomic status (SES) (See Fitzgerald et al., 2000; Zucker, et al. 1996). AALs not only provide a higher risk environment with respect to psychopathology and poor social adaptation, but also are downwardly socially mobile relative to their own parents, live in families with higher levels of family violence, and have higher rates of separation and divorce. Moreover, familial risk structure tends to cumulate across generations. Fuller et al. (2003) identified two critical intergenerational pathways of risk. One pathway involved the transmission of aggression (marital conflict, antisocial behavior, parent-child conflict) across two generations (grandparent to parent). The second pathway, unique to men, involved alcoholism: grandfather alcoholism was related to fathers' alcoholism and behavior problems, which in turn was related to sons' aggression. Thus, evidence from the MLS strongly characterizes the parental rearing environment as risk loaded, and children reared in such environments are more vulnerable to poor developmental outcomes. The most reasonable hypothesis concerning child outcomes, therefore, is that children reared in such environments will reflect the parental and familial dysfunction to which they are exposed. We have found this to be especially true for children reared in AAL families.

CHARACTERISTICS OF CHILDREN:
PRESCHOOL TO ELEMENTARY AGES

Cross-sectional comparisons at ages 3-5 showed that, in general, COAs have higher levels of hyperactivity, more negative mood, more problematic social relationships, greater deficits in cognitive functioning, higher levels of aggressive behavior, and more precocious acquisition of cognitive schemas about alcohol and other drugs than children from control families (Poon et al., 2000; Zucker et al., 2000; Zucker et al., 1995b). Consistent with the risk aggregation conceptual framework, we found that developmental risk was elevated in families where both parents had an alcohol use disorder, or where at least one parent met criteria for antisocial personality disorder in addition to the alcohol problems (Mun, Fitzgerald, von Eye, Puttler & Zucker, 2001). Children in these families with higher parental psychopathology were more distractable and reactive compared to children in families with lower parental psychopathology. Moreover, child risky temperament appeared to be nested in suboptimal rearing environments. The Mun et al. findings indicate that child temperament, externalizing and internalizing problem behavior, and parental psychopathology are highly interrelated and aggregate and intensify risk structure (consistent with predictions from our conceptual framework). Specifically, this study demonstrated that each of four dimensions of temperament were associated with higher levels of behavior problems; activity, distractability, and reactivity were related to externalizing behavior, whereas withdrawal was related to internalizing behavior.

Although there are many theories about temperament, since the early 20th century it is generally believed to be a component of personality that is strongly influenced by biological factors (genetic and/or congenital in origin) (Strelau, 1998). Some components of personality endure (continuity) and others change over the life course (discontinuity) as a result of the complex gene-environment transactions that characterize human development (Gottlieb, 1991; Yates, Egeland & Sroufe, 2003). The findings from Mun et al. suggest that dimensions of temperament not only provide evidence of individual differences among the COAs in the MLS, but also present the possibility that temperamental variation may contribute to variations in child development, particularly within the context of parent-child interactions.

What other factors are involved in the risk structure models that we are assessing? Loukas, Piejak, Bingham, Fitzgerald and Zucker (2001) found that parental alcohol problems and antisocial behavior were associated with elevated rates of parental health problems (illnesses and hospitalizations) and distress, as well as to child behavior problems. Specifically, parental distress accounted for the relationship between alcohol related psychopathology and health and behavior problems. However, there was also a direct relationship between parental alcoholism and antisocial behavior problems in preschool age children. Loukas, Fitzgerald, Zucker and von Eye (2001) examined this finding further by assessing how parental alcoholism and antisocial behavior affected externalizing behavior problems. They found that family conflict and father-son conflict accounted for the relationship between parental antisocial behavior effects on child externalizing behavior and that child lack of control mediated parental alcoholism effects. The mediational role of family conflict was consistent across both maternal and paternal models; that is, higher lifetime antisocial behavior of parents during the preschool years predicted child externalizing behavior during the early elementary years. However, the strongest predictor of externalizing behavior during the early elementary years was the child's own externalizing behavior during the preschool years. This autostability is most likely attributable to difficult temperament, present from the infancy-toddler period, and to the high stress environments in which children are reared (Zucker & Wong, 2005).

A number of studies have demonstrated that highly undercontrolled children tend to retain rankings in levels of undercontrol over time. Although externalizing behavior problems tend to decrease throughout the elementary years, the rate of decline is not the same for all children. Consistent with Mun et al. (2001), boys showed fewer disruptive behavior problems as they grew older, but retained their rank order over a six-year period (Loukas, Zucker, Fitzgerald & Krull, 2003). Moreover, some boys maintained high levels of disruptive behavior, possibly elevating their risk for maladaptive behavior and psychopathology during the adolescent years. One might expect that children with high levels of behavior problems and slow or nonexistent rates of decline would be at maximum risk for early onset of drinking and other risk behaviors, and this does appear to be the case.

PATHWAYS TO EARLY ONSET

Mayzer, Puttler, Fitzgerald and Zucker (2002) scanned the longitudinal sample and identified children who reported their first drink prior to age 14 (First Drinkers) and those who had not (No First Drinkers). Because the MLS is a prospective study, they were able to then connect

First Drinkers' and No First Drinkers' characteristics from the pre-school years to their early or no onset drinking status during early ado-lescence. The investigators set out to answer two questions. First, do early drinkers demonstrate stronger continuity in external behavior problems from preschool through adolescence? Second, if these conti-nuity differences are present, what are the key mediators of the stronger continuity characteristic of First Drinkers? We found that first drinkers, as preschoolers, were more likely to have both externalizing (cruel to animals, lie, set fires, destroy things) and internalizing (sad, depressed, worried) behaviors than were No First Drinkers. In addition, First Drink-ers were more often reported to be immature, overweight, nervous, to express "strange ideas," and to have trouble sleeping. At school age, teachers were more likely to attribute behavior problems to First Drink-ers than to No First Drinkers. During adolescence, First Drinkers were more likely to be associated with delinquent peers and peers who had been detained by the police, been in juvenile court and spent time in jail. In addition, Mayzer et al. found that First Drinkers were less likely to be involved with conventional activities, such as participation in athletics, school plays, and band, or to attend a religious service at least once a month or more.

Wong and her colleagues (Wong, Brower, Fitzgerald & Zucker, 2004) examined one of the possible mediators identified by Mayzer et al. (2002), sleep disturbance, to determine whether it might provide an early warn-ing sign of biobehavioral dysregulation. They noted that insomnia often is linked with alcoholism among adults. Wong et al. found that children reported to have sleep problems during the preschool period were more likely to use alcohol, marijuana, and other drugs during late childhood and early adolescence. Sleep problems also increased the risk for early onset of occasional or regular cigarette use. Other predictors of early use (such as attention problems, anxiety/depression, and aggression) in late childhood did not attenuate the relationship between sleep mea-sures and substance use.

The studies by Mayzer et al. (2002) and Wong et al. (2004) provide strong support for the hypothesis that markers of adolescent alcohol and other drug use, as well as more general biobehavioral dysregulation can be detected very early in the life course. Moreover, they provide addi-tional support for continuity models of etiology with respect to the development of substance abuse disorders as well as co-occurring psychopathology.

Evidence for continuity in biobehavioral dysregulation, however, is not the only indicator of early risk. There is also evidence that very early in development, COAs begin to develop cognitive structures or schemas about alcohol and that they associate these schemas with expectancies about the effects of alcohol as well as the role of alcohol in adult behavior (Fitzgerald, Puttler, Mun & Zucker, 2000).

Findings regarding early cognitive schemas about alcohol use are particularly disturbing because they suggest that very early in development, children are forming conceptual frameworks about their relation to the world that incorporate the intergenerational dynamics identified by Fuller et al. (2003). The emergence of alcohol-related schemas is of particular concern because they indicate that emergent behavioral and cognitive disorganization is being supported by underlying deep structure mental models or expectancies that shape the individual's self-identity and self-other relationships in the context of family substance abuse and disorganization (Zucker et al., 1995). For example, preschool-age sons of male alcoholics are better able to identify specific alcoholic beverages and to correctly identify a larger number of alcoholic beverages than are sons of nonalcoholics. These data indicate that the children's cognitive schemas include alcohol consumption as an attribute associated with being male, and are associated with specific parental roles. These emergent schemas may also incorporate emotional components related to high marital and family conflict into an emergent autobiographical memory of family alcohol events that may subsequently influence peer selection and romantic relationships when they become relevant life course experiences (Fitzgerald et al., 2000).

Thus, as early as the preschool years, sons of alcoholics have organized a system of dysfunctional behaviors, cognitions, and self-concepts that are symptomatic of psychopathology and that are embedded within the maintenance structures of poor parenting, poor family relationships and poor socioeconomic resources. A critical question for prevention efforts concerns the extent to which the child's behavior is context specific, or whether it generalizes to other settings. If such behavior is specific to the home environment, then prevention efforts can be tailor made to the home setting and to the family dynamics that promote and maintain behavior problems and risk for substance abuse. If such behaviors generalize to other contexts, a broader set of prevention efforts would be required in order to impact significant components of the risk system necessary to move the child from a high risk pathway to a low risk pathway. School is one of the most important contexts outside the home because children spend so much time there daily, and because it provides the course for development of many peer networks. So we enlisted teachers as part of our data collection team and asked them to assess children's behavior problems, school achievement, general social status, as well as the level of interest parents seem to show in their child's school experience. Our findings support the broader model. For example, teachers' descriptions of children's behavior were consistent with the AAL, NAAL and Control groupings, even though these groupings were completely unknown to the teachers. Although teacher ratings of child aggression, activity, like-ability, and attractiveness did not statistically differentiate the groups, the means were in the expected direction with AAL children rated lowest. When asked to forecast child performance in middle school, elementary teachers projected the poorest school performance for AAL children. Teacher reports also indicated that AAL parents showed less interest in their children's school performance than NAAL or Control parents (see Fitzgerald et al., 2002). This finding is particularly important from a prevention perspective because the general literature clearly indicates a positive effect on children's performance when parents are involved with schools and negative effects when they are not (Hill et al., 2004). Finally, differences in behavioral regulation and social competence are mirrored by differences in academic performance: sons of AALS do more poorly than do sons of NAALS or controls (Poon et al., 2000).

A PERSON CENTERED APPROACH TO RISK AND RESILIENCE

Recently, Zucker and his colleagues developed models to assess etiologic issues related to risk and resilience, where resilience was defined as a successful adaptation to life circumstances despite adversity generated by the rearing environment (Zucker, Wong, Puttler & Fitzgerald, 2003). Their goal was to identify individual characteristics and aspects of the rearing environment that relate to positive developmental outcomes. A family adversity index was developed that scaled parental psychopathology, taking into account both the currency and the severity of parental alcohol use disorder among both parents, as well as the presence or absence of parental antisocial behavior. The child's adaptation was characterized by a global sociobehavioral psychopathology index. This strategy allowed the investigators to characterize four types of children: *Resilient* children were defined as those with high adaptation in the context of high family adversity; *Nonchallenged* children were defined as having normal adaptation under conditions of low family adversity; *Vulnerable* children experienced low adaptation (high psychopathology) under conditions of high family adversity; *Troubled* children experienced high psychopathology under conditions of low adversity (indicating they had poor behavioral adaptation even without significant family adversity; see Zucker et al., 2003).

Nonchallenged children had the lowest level of externalizing behavior problems followed in order by the resilient, troubled, and vulnerable children. At all ages, vulnerable children had the highest level of externalizing behavior and were significantly different from the least challenged group. Although resilient children were not different from their nonchallenged peers as preschoolers, they consistently showed a slightly higher level of externalizing behavior as they grew older.

Nonchallenged children also had the lowest levels of internalizing behavior problems, followed by the resilient children. During preschool and the early elementary years, nonchallenged and resilient children had fewer internalizing symptoms than either vulnerable or troubled children, However, by early adolescence, the nonchallenged group was significantly lower than all other groups with the resilient children showing a rise in internalizing behavior to the same level seen in the vulnerable and troubled children by ages 12-14. Thus, by early adolescence, vulnerable children were at highest risk, the nonchallenged children were at lowest risk, and the resilient children were at intermediary risk, particularly because of the increase in internalizing symptoms during puberty.

This person centered approach will provide increasing insight into the nested elements that structure both continuous and discontinuous risk pathways characterizing the development of alcohol use disorders. The key will be to link the relationships among biological, social, psychological and ecological variables to explicit prevention efforts that are tailored to the degrees of vulnerability to which children of alcoholics are exposed.

EMERGENT PATHWAYS: STRUCTURING RISK AGGREGATION

Summing over the 18 years of longitudinal data collected to date, findings from the MLS suggest that there are at least three developmental pathways characterizing the children in the study. One pathway describes strong continuity across at least a 15 year span, and reflects the early emergence of maladaptive behavior that is supported by familial, neighborhood, and peer maintenance structures sufficient to organize biobehavioral dysregulation as a life-course pathway (Fitzgerald et al., 2000).

In this pathway, high biobehavioral dysregulation during preschool (difficult temperament, externalizing behavior, poor cognitive functioning), is maintained during the elementary years, then expressed during adolescence by early onset drinking, smoking, and active sexual behavior, poor school performance, and involvement with the criminal justice system. This pathway is most likely to characterize children reared in AAL families.

The other two pathways are marked by greater discontinuity, with strong individual differences and greater heterogeneity in the actions of both risk and protective factors (Zucker, Chermack & Curran, 2000; Zucker, 2003). The preschool and childhood periods for children on these pathways are essentially identical. However, it is during middle childhood that differentiation begins, as family disorganization, conflict, unemployment, and perhaps, divorce increase, and the pathways through adolescence become dynamically bound to experiential variations in adversity as well as underlying biological variation. These pathways reflect the broader heterogeneity of characteristics among NAAL families.

CONCLUSIONS

The findings we have summarized in this article represent only a sample of results from the Michigan Longitudinal Study of children at risk for alcoholism and co-occurring psychopathology. Findings were drawn primarily from studies involving the first 4 waves of data collection (child ages from 3 to 14). To date we have identified three major pathways of risk; one a strong continuity pathway, and two discontinuous pathways. The two types of pathways suggest different prevention strategies. The strong continuity pathway has it origins at least as far back as the preschool years and is more likely to characterize children reared in antisocial alcoholic families. Prevention efforts for these children are likely to be maximally effective if they begin during the infant and toddler years, with a focus on reducing family dynamics (conflict, aggression) that both induce and maintain dysfunctional behavior in children. Because children traveling strong continuity pathways also are at high risk for genetic and inter-generational risks, prevention efforts most likely will also have to be available over much of childhood in order to inoculate against and counter persistent risk. In contrast, prevention programs targeting children on discontinuous pathways are likely to be more successful even when the prevention efforts are tied to specific transitional periods or events in development that induce vulnerability. Such events may include transition from elementary school to middle school (exposure to new peer group, isolation from group), significant changes in the family (divorce, death, loss of employment), or the substantive personal changes that accompany puberty. Clearly, stronger bridges need to be built to link etiologic research with prevention research if we are to meaningfully reduce the impact of alcoholism on child development.

REFERENCES

Carmichael Olson, H., O'Connor, M. J., & Fitzgerald, H. E. (2001). Lessons learned from study of the developmental impact of parental alcoholism. *Infant Mental Health Journal, 22,* 271-290.

Fitzgerald, H. E., Davies, W. H., & Zucker, R. A. (Eds.), (2002). Growing up in an alcoholic family: Structuring pathways for risk aggregation and theory-driven intervention. In R. MacMahon & R. deV. Peters (Eds.). *30th Banff Conference on Behaviour Science, Children of disordered parents* (pp. 127-146). Boston, Kluwer.

Fitzgerald, H. E., Davies, W. H., Zucker, R. A., & Klinger, M. (1994). Developmental systems theory and substance abuse: a conceptual and methodological framework for analyzing patterns of variation in families. In L.L'Abate (Ed.), *Handbook of developmental family psychology and psychopathology* (pp. 350-372). New York: Wiley.

Fitzgerald, H. E., Puttler, L. I., Mun, E. Y., & Zucker, R. A. (2000). Prenatal and postnatal exposure to parental alcohol use and abuse. In J. D. Osofsky & H. E. Fitzgerald (Eds.), *WAIMH handbook of infant mental health: Vol. 4. Infant mental health in groups at risk* (pp. 123-159). New York: Wiley.

Fitzgerald, H. E., Zucker, R. A., & Yang, H-Y. (1995). Developmental systems theory and alcoholism: Analyzing patterns of variation in high risk families. *Psychology of Addictive Behaviors, 9,* 8-22.

Fitzgerald, H. E., Zucker, R. A., Puttler, L. I., Caplan, H. M., & Mun, E.-Y. (2000). Alcohol abuse/dependence in women and girls: aetiology, course, and subtype variations. *Alcoscope: International review of alcohol management, 3*(1), 6-10.

Fuller, E., Chermack, S. T., Cruise, K. A., Kirsch, E., Fitzgerald, H. E., & Zucker, R. A. (2003). Predictors of childhood aggression across three generations in children of alcoholics: Relationships involving parental alcoholism, individual and spousal and aggression, and parenting practices. *Journal of Studies on Alcohol, 64,* 472-483.

Grant, B. F. (2000). Estimates of U. S. Children exposed to alcohol abuse and dependence in the family. *American Journal of Public Health, 90,* 112-115.

Grant, B. F., & Dawson, D. A. (1997). Age of onset of alcohol use and its association with DSM-IV alcohol abuse and dependence: Results from the National Longitudinal Alcohol Epidemiologic Survey. *Journal of Substance Abuse, 9,* 103-110.

Gottlieb, G. (1991). Experiential canalization of behavior development: theory. *Developmental Psychology, 27,* 4-13.

Hill, N. E., Castellino, D. R., Lansford, J. E., Nowlin, P., Dodge, K. A., Bates, J. E., & Pettit, G. S. (2004). Parent academic involvement as related to school behavior, achievement, and aspirations: Demographic variations across adolescence. *Child Development, 75,* 1491-1509.

Ichiyama, M. A., Zucker, R. A., Fitzgerald, H. E, & Bingham, C. R. (1996). Articulating subtype differences in self and relational experience among alcoholic men via structural analysis of social behavior. *Journal of Consulting and Clinical Psychology, 64,* 1245-1254.

Jester, J. M., Zucker, R. A., Wong, M. M., & Fitzgerald, H. E. (2000). Marital assortment in high-risk population (Abstract). *Alcoholism: Clinical and Experimental Research, 24,* Supplement, 36A.

Loukas, A., Fitzgerald, H. E., Zucker, R. A., & von Eye. A. (2001). Alcohol problems and antisocial behavior: Relations to externalizing behavior problems among young sons. *Journal of Abnormal Child Psychology, 29,* 91-106.

Loukas, A., Zucker, R. A., Fitzgerald, H. E., & Krull, J. (2003). Developmental trajectories of disruptive behavior problems among sons of alcoholics: Effects of parent psychopathology, family conflict, and child under control. *Journal of Abnormal Psychology, 112,* 119-131.

Loukas, A., Piejak, L. A., Bingham, C. R., Fitzgerald, H. E., & Zucker, R. A. (2001). Parental distress as a mediator of child problem outcomes in alcoholic families. *Family Relations: Interdisciplinary Journal of Family Studies, 50,* 293-301.

Mayzer, R., Puttler, L. I., Fitzgerald, H. E., & Zucker, R. A. (2002). Predicting early onset of first alcohol use from behavior problem indicators in early childhood. *Alcoholism: Clinical and Experimental Research, 26,* 124A.

McAweeney, M. J., Zucker, R. A., Fitzgerald, H. E., Puttler, L., Wong, M. M. (2005). Individual and partner predictors of recovery from Alcohol Use Disorder over a nine-year interval: Findings from a community sample of alcoholic married men. *Journal of Studies on Alcohol, 66,* 220-228.

Mun, E-Y., Fitzgerald, H. E., Puttler, L. I., Zucker, R. A., & von Eye, A. (2001). Temperamental characteristics as predictors of externalizing and internalizing child behavior problems in the contexts of high and low parental psychopathology. *Infant Mental Health Journal, 22,* 393-415.

Poon, E., Ellis, D. A., Fitzgerald, H. E., & Zucker, R. A. (2000). Cognitive functioning of sons of alcoholics during the early elementary school years: Differences related to subtypes of familial alcoholism. *Alcoholism: Clinical and Experimental Research, 23,* 1020-1027.

SAMHSA (1998). Preliminary results from the 1997 National Household Survey on Drug Abuse. (DHHS Publications Document No. SMA 98-3251). Rockville, MD.

Strelau, J. (1998). *Temperament: A psychological perspective.* New York: Plenum Press.

Tarter, R. E., & Vanukov, M. M. (1994). Alcoholism: A developmental disorder. *Journal of Consulting and Clinical Psychology, 62,* 1096-1106.

Wong, M. M., Brower, K. J., Fitzgerald, H. E., & Zucker, R. A. (2004). Sleep problems in childhood and early onset of alcohol and other drug use in adolescence. *Alcoholism: Clinical and Experimental Research, 28,* 578-587.

Yates, T. M., Egeland, B., & Sroufe, L. A. (2003). Rethinking resilience: A developmental process perspective. In S. S. Luthar (Ed.), *Resilience and vulnerability: Adaptation in the context of childhood adversity* (pp. 243-266). New York: Cambridge University Press.

Zucker, R. A. (1987). The four alcoholisms: a developmental account of the etiologic process. In P. C. Rivers (Ed.), *Alcohol and Addictive Behaviors Nebraska Symposium on Motivation* (pp. 27-83). Lincoln, NE: University of Nebraska Press.

Zucker, R.A. (1989). Is risk for alcoholism predictable? A probabilistic approach to a developmental problem. *Drugs and Society, 4,* 69-93.

Zucker, R. A. (2003, October). *Risk for addictive disorders early in life: New findings, new models of prevention.* Invited address at the American Society for Addiction Medicine (ASAM), Washington, D.C.

Zucker, R. A. (In press). Alcohol use and the Alcohol Use Disorders: A developmental biopsychosocial formulation covering the life course. In Cicchetti, D. & Cohen, D. J. (Eds.) *Developmental psychopathology (2nd ed.).* New York: Wiley.

Zucker, R.A., Chermack, S.T., & Curran, G. M. (2000). Alcoholism: A lifespan perspective on etiology and course. In Sameroff, A., Lewis, M., & Miller, S. (Eds.), *Handbook of Developmental Psychopathology* (2nd Ed.) (pp. 569-587). New York: Plenum.

Zucker, R. A., Ellis, D. A., & Fitzgerald, H. E. (1994). Developmental evidence for at least two alcoholisms: I. Biopsychosoocial variation among pathways into symptomatic difficulty. *Annals of the New York Academy of Science, 708,* 134-146.

Zucker, R. A., Ellis, D. A., Bingham, C. R., Fitzgerald, H. E., & Sanford, K. P. (1996). Other evidence for at least two alcoholisms, II: Life course variation in antisociality and heterogeneity of alcoholic outcome. *Development and Psychopathology, 8,* 831-848.

Zucker, R. A., & Fitzgerald, H. E. (1991). Early developmental factors and risk for alcohol problems. *Alcohol Health & Research World, 15,* 18-24.

Zucker, R. A., Fitzgerald, H. E., & Moses, H. (1995a). Emergence of alcohol problems and the several alcoholisms: A developmental perspective on etiologic theory and life course trajectory. In D. Cicchetti & D. Cohen (Eds.), *Manual of Developmental Psychopathology* Vol 2: *Risk, disorder, and adaptation* (pp. 677-711). New York: Wiley.

Zucker, R. A., Fitzgerald, H. E., Refior, S. K., Puttler, L. I., Pallas, D. M., & Ellis, D. A. (2000). The clinical and social ecology of childhood for children of alcoholics: Description of a study and implications for a differentiated social policy. In H. E. Fitzgerald, B. M.. Lester, & B. Zuckerman (Eds.), *Children of addiction: Research, health, and public policy issues* (pp. 109-141). New York: Garland.

Zucker, R. A., Kincaid, S. B., Fitzgerald, H. E., & Bingham, C. R. (1995b). Alcohol schema acquisition in preschoolers: Differences between COAs and non-COAs. *Alcoholism: Clinical and Experimental Research, 19,* 1011-1017.

Zucker, R. A., & Wong, M. M. (2005). Prevention for children of alcoholics and other high risk groups. In M. Galanter (Ed.), *Recent developments in alcoholism. Vol. XVII. Research on alcohol problems in adolescents and young adults.* (Ch. 14, pp. 299-319). New York: Kluwer Academic/Plenum.

Zucker, R. A., Wong, M. M., Puttler, L. I., & Fitzgerald, H. E. (2003). Resilience and vulnerability among sons of alcoholics: Relationship to developmental outcomes between early childhood and adolescence. In S. Luthar (Ed.), *Resilience and vulnerability* (pp. 76-103). New York: Cambridge University Press.

doi:10.1300/J020v25n01_02

Family Response to Adolescence, Youth and Alcohol

Judith L. Fischer, PhD
Boyd W. Pidcock, PhD
Barbra J. Fletcher-Stephens, PhD

SUMMARY. This review highlights three aspects of adolescent alcohol use and misuse that have ramifications for families: (a) adolescent disinhibition, (b) substance-specific parenting factors, and (c) non-substance-specific parenting factors. Although there are a great number of adolescent treatment models currently utilized across the country, this review focuses on three integrated family-based treatment models with proven efficacy: (a) Multisystemic Therapy (MST; Henggeler, Schoenwald, Borduin, Rawland, & Cunningham, 1998), (b) Brief Strategic Family Therapy (BSFT; Szapocznik, Hervis, & Schwartz, 2003), and (c) Multidimensional

---

Judith L. Fischer is affiliated with Dept. of Human Development and Family Studies at Texas Tech University, Lubbock, TX 79409 (E-mail: Judith.fischer@ttu.edu).

Boyd W. Pidcock is Program Coordinator of the Addictions Studies Program, Department of Counseling Psychology, CB 86, Lewis & Clark College, Portland, OR 97219 (E-mail: pidcock@lclark.edu).

Barbra J. Fletcher-Stephens is Director of African American Family Studies Program in the Department of Marriage, Family and Children Counseling, Pacific Oaks College, Pasadena, CA (E-mail: bfletcher-stephens@pacificoaks.edu).

[Haworth co-indexing entry note]: "Family Response to Adolescence, Youth and Alcohol." Fischer, Judith L., Boyd W. Pidcock, and Barbra J. Fletcher-Stephens. Co-published simultaneously in *Alcoholism Treatment Quarterly* (The Haworth Press, Inc.) Vol. 25, No. 1/2, 2007, pp. 27-41; and: *Familial Responses to Alcohol Problems* (ed: Judith L. Fischer, Miriam Mulsow, and Alan W. Korinek) The Haworth Press, Inc., 2007, pp. 27-41. Single or multiple copies of this article are available for a fee from The Haworth Document Delivery Service [1-800-HAWORTH, 9:00 a.m. - 5:00 p.m. (EST). E-mail address: docdelivery@haworthpress.com].

Family Therapy (MDFT; Liddle, 2004; Center for Substance Abuse Treatment [CSAT], 2004). These family-based therapies focus on accurately assessing multiple influences and targeting effective intervention strategies designed to support changes throughout a number of systems that affect and serve to reinforce or support the adolescent's problem behaviors. doi:10.1300/J020v25n01_03 *[Article copies available for a fee from The Haworth Document Delivery Service: 1-800-HAWORTH. E-mail address: <docdelivery@haworthpress.com> Website: <http://www.HaworthPress.com> © 2007 by The Haworth Press, Inc. All rights reserved.]*

KEYWORDS. Adolescent alcohol use, parenting factors, adolescent treatment

INTRODUCTION

A biopsychosocial approach to the study of alcohol and families (Zucker, Boyd, & Howard, 1994) organizes the prediction of pathological alcohol involvement through consideration of (a) biological contributions such as genetic vulnerability and resilience, (b) psychological factors including perception, cognition, expectancy, emotion, personality, and behavior, and (c) social influences such as parenting, peer influences, social settings, and cultural messages. The focus in this review is on family response to adolescents and youth and alcohol. Because adolescents often use and abuse alcohol together with other substances, such research is included in this review. We consider research within the framework of the biopsychosocial model and highlight intervention to ameliorate family and adolescent problems with adolescent alcohol use and misuse.

RESEARCH ON ADOLESCENT ALCOHOL USE AND MISUSE AND FAMILIES

The period of adolescence in North America, roughly ages 13 to 19, is characterized by dramatic increases in substance use. The Monitoring the Future's annual national survey reported in 2003 that 20% of eighth graders acknowledged having been drunk in their lifetimes, but almost three times as many twelfth graders indicated having been drunk (58%) (Johnston, O'Malley, Bachman, & Schulenberg, 2003). The period of youth or emerging adulthood, ages 18 to 25, reflects peak substance use and abuse (National Institute on Alcohol Abuse and Alcoholism, 2000).

An important advance in the explanation of adolescent alcohol use and misuse considers the identification of both mediating and moderating effects (Fischer & Lyness, 2005). Mediating effects describe how a process may work; moderating effects specify for whom and under what conditions associations hold between and among variables (Sher, 1994). This review highlights three aspects of adolescent alcohol use and misuse that have ramifications for families: (a) adolescent disinhibition, (b) substance-specific parenting factors, and (c) non-substance-specific parenting factors. Although the biopsychosocial model includes more factors than covered by this limited list, a review of these three aspects aids in the understanding of families and adolescent alcohol use.

Adolescent Disinhibition

The role of disinhibition has gathered research attention as a factor in adolescent substance use and abuse (Iacono, Carlson, Taylor, Elkins, & McGue, 1999). Characteristics of disinhibition related to substance use include impulsive sensation seeking and aggression (Zuckerman & Kuhlman, 2000), poor behavioral self-control (Wills & Dishion, 2004), behavioral problems (Barnow, Schuckit, & Lucht, 2002), and delinquency (Bui, Ellickson, & Bell, 2000). Barnow et al.'s (2002) research on German adolescents described the characteristics of adolescents with alcohol problems: they had more behavioral problems, more perceived parental rejection, less parental warmth, and more association with substance-using peers than did adolescents without alcohol problems. Those adolescents described as alcoholic demonstrated all of the characteristics plus aggression/delinquency.

Substance-Specific Parenting Factors

A family history of alcoholism (a substance-specific parenting factor) is an important element in adolescent development of substance use problems (Jacob & Johnson, 1997). But findings have been inconsistent from study to study (Fischer & Wampler, 1994). Substance abuse in children can, and does, occur in families without parental alcoholism (Pandina & Johnson, 1990). In families with parental alcohol use and abuse, children develop expectancies and imitative behaviors (Sher, 1994), but parental recovery does not necessarily correlate with reduced offspring substance use (Pidcock & Fischer, 1998). The timing of exposure to parental substance use disorders is important. Although childhood exposure conferred a nonsignificant risk on offspring, adolescent exposure was associated with a threefold significant risk for the emergence of substance use disorders (Biederman, Faraone, Monuteaux, & Feighner, 2000).

The mechanism by which parental substance use confers risks may be direct or indirect. Adolescents may use substances themselves to reduce or numb the negative emotional states they experience in the face of parental alcohol abuse (Sher, 1994), one example of a direct effect. A mediating effect occurs when the associations between parental alcoholism and offspring substance use are accounted for, in part or in full, by a third variable. For example, family addictions are related to family dysfunction that is, in turn, related to offspring alcohol misuse (Wampler, Fischer, Thomas, & Lyness, 1993). A substance using older sibling models use or provides substances for a younger child in the family (Duncan, Duncan & Hops, 1996). Duncan et al. (1996) concluded that parents' substance use effects on younger sibling's use were indirect and operated through the effects of the parents on older sibling's use. With children from the "same" alcoholic or dysfunctional family experiencing different outcomes, more research is needed on siblings (cf., Fischer, Pidcock, Munsch, & Forthun, 2005).

Moderating factors that have been found to alter the association between parental drinking and offspring outcomes include expectations (VanVoorst & Quirk, 2003), family cohesion (Farrell, Barnes, & Banerjee, 1995), and personality of the offspring (Fischer & Wampler, 1994). Fischer and Wampler (1994) found that personality was a moderator of the association of family addictions with offspring drinking for both males and females, but family roles were moderators only with respect to family dysfunction. The research of Farrell et al. (1995) indicated that family cohesion buffered adolescents against the impacts of paternal drinking. Although a good parent-child relationship is important to positive child adjustment, it may not always be protective in situations in which parents use substances (Andrews, Hops, & Duncan, 1997).

King and Chassin's (2004) research tested for both mediators and moderators of the link between parental alcoholism and offspring substance use disorders in emerging adults (ages 18-25). Their longitudinal study included measures of adolescent undercontrol. The mediation results suggested that children of alcoholics (COAs) have greater drug use disorder risks in emerging adulthood due to their own undercontrol as well as their parent's inconsistent discipline. Among adolescents with lower levels of behavioral undercontrol, but not among those with higher levels, parental support had a buffering or moderating effect on drug use in emerging adulthood.

Non-Substance-Specific Parenting Factors

Supervision and support (non-substance-specific parenting factors) are important parenting variables that operate regardless of parental substance use or abuse to influence adolescent outcomes (Jacob & Johnson, 1997). Abstaining adolescents have parents who do not use punishment to maintain control but instead clarify appropriate behavior and reinforce that behavior; such parents also have warm relationships with their children (Coombs & Landsverk, 1988). Active parental monitoring is essential. That is, parents should structure "the child's home, school, and community environments...[in ways that are] developmentally, contextually, and culturally appropriate" (Dishion & McMahon, 1998, p. 66).

Some scholars have theorized that single-parent family structure creates problems for adolescents that may lead to their greater substance experimentation and abuse. Jeynes's (2001) research of U.S. twelfth graders found that adolescents who had experienced more recent parental divorce drank more alcohol. But Curry, Fischer, Reifman, and Harris (2004) reported that the association between parental divorce and adolescent alcohol use was mediated by other variables, including parent unavailability, family quality, peer acceptance/self-esteem, and deviant peer involvement.

Regardless of intactness of family of origin, parental support is an important main effect of adolescent alcohol use, but it is also mediated by other factors. According to Bogenschneider, Wu, and Raffaelli (1998), mothers' responsiveness acted indirectly on adolescent alcohol use by helping to weaken adolescents' orientation to peers. In addition, Wills and Cleary (1996) suggested that parent support buffers or moderates adolescent substance use by reducing the effects of risk factors and increasing the effects of protective factors. The combination of supervision and acceptance, termed authoritative parenting style, has been identified as a particularly important factor, both concurrently and longitudinally, in the reduced use of substances (Adalbjarnardottir & Hafsteinsson, 2001).

In addition to parenting style, the quality of parent-child communication is also important. Kafka and London (1991) established the value of an adolescent's having at least one parent with whom the adolescent has "open" communication (as opposed to closed or neither open nor closed communication). They found reduced levels of substance use among high school–aged adolescents who had such a parent. What and when parents tell their children about substance use and abuse is pivotal.

Ennett, Bauman, Foshee, Pemberton, and Hicks (2001) discovered that, for adolescents who were already using substances, parent-child communication on rules and discipline actually made the situation worse. Parents should begin communicating with their children about substance use before the children begin use.

Whether initiated by parents, or located in parents' responses to events, trauma is another pathway to adolescent problem behavior. Adolescents in substance abuse treatment programs have reported more physical, sexual, and violent victimization compared with controls (National Institute on Alcohol Abuse and Alcoholism, 1997). The dual risks of COA status and sexual abuse in adolescence have been related to higher levels of adolescent problems, including chemical abuse, than that found in adolescents with only one risk factor (Chandy, Blum, & Resnick, 1996). Adolescents experiencing current abuse reported more problem behaviors, such as binge drinking, than adolescents with histories of prior abuse (Luster & Small, 1997). Research indicates that the impact of victimization can be ameliorated by a very supportive relationship with a parent and by close parental monitoring of adolescent behavior (Luster & Small, 1997).

In sum, difficulties in making the transition from childhood to adolescence are compounded when alcohol and drugs enter the picture. Parent's use of substances gains added importance as a source of information and modeling and as a stressor in the family. Support and monitoring are possible mediators and buffers for adolescents. Variations in these processes across families and variations within families may explain the varying outcomes of adolescents.

FAMILY-BASED ADOLESCENT TREATMENT

The focus of this section is limited to providing a general overview of key issues relevant to family-based treatment models currently utilized for adolescent alcohol and substance abuse and dependency. Although, in general, the adolescent treatment field is relatively young and under-researched (Grella, Joshi, & Hser, 2004), during the last decade family-based therapies have been developed and proliferated and represent the most thoroughly researched treatment modality for adolescent substance use (Liddle, 2004). Importantly, the research has consistently indicated that specific integrated family-based therapy models offer innovative and effective treatment for adolescent substance use (Drug Strategies, 2002; Grella et al., 2004; Kaminer, 2001; Liddle, 2004).

Although there are a great number of adolescent treatment models currently utilized across the country, this review focuses on three integrated family-based treatment models with proven efficacy: (a) Multisystemic Therapy (MST; Henggeler, Schoenwald, Borduin, Rawland, & Cunningham, 1998), (b) Brief Strategic Family Therapy (BSFT; Szapocznik, Hervis, & Schwartz, 2003), and (c) Multidimensional Family Therapy (MDFT; Liddle, 2004; Center for Substance Abuse Treatment [CSAT], 2004).

Adolescent Treatment Issues

The review of the literature on adolescent alcohol and substance use elaborates an array of biopsychosocial factors across individual, family, peer, and community levels. Many adolescent substance users experience significant negative consequences requiring intervention and treatment. However, current figures tend to indicate that treatment availability is scarce for adolescents in need compared to similar services for adults. For example, Kaminer (2001) cites regional studies that report as many as 7-10% of substance using adolescents may be in need of treatment while very few actually receive help, often only those most severely impacted with comorbid psychiatric problems or those entering treatment through the criminal justice system. A recent national study drawn from 23 adolescent drug treatment programs (Grella et al., 2004; Riggs, 2003) found that 64% of adolescents in substance abuse treatment had at least one Diagnostic and Statistical Manual of Mental Disorders-IV (DSM-IV-TR; American Psychiatric Association, 2000) diagnosable mental health disorder. Of the adolescents diagnosed with a mental health disorder, 59% were diagnosed with conduct disorder, 15% with depression, and 13% with attention-deficit hyperactivity disorder (Foxhall, 2001). Further support for the paucity of treatment availability for adolescents is documented by the National Household Survey on Drug Abuse (2002). The 2001 survey reported that 1.1 million youths between the ages of 12-17 needed treatment for alcohol and substance misuse but, of those, only approximately 10% actually received services. The limited availability of adolescent-specific substance abuse treatment is generally credited to limited resources, an historical focus on individual-level adult treatment, and lack of a clear consensus on evidence-based treatment strategies (Kaminer, 2001).

In summary, the research clearly indicates that a significant percentage of American adolescents are currently experiencing alcohol and substance abuse and related problems and are in need of immediate treatment services. Additionally, the problems of the adolescents are occurring across multiple domains of the adolescents' functioning and the worlds in which they are embedded. These complex problems are not confined to the narrow dimension of alcohol or substance abuse. Today's adolescents are impacted and influenced by the complex interactions of micro level risk as well as macro level risks found within themselves, their families, their peer-groups, and their communities (Drug Strategies, 2002; Foxhall, 2001; Grella et al., 2004).

What Works in Adolescent Treatment

Given that adolescent treatment is relatively new, so, too, is evaluation research examining adolescent treatment model efficacy (Drug Strategies, 2002; Liddle, 2004). Historically, the vast majority of research funding has been dedicated to evaluating adult treatment services (Grella et al., 2004). The small numbers of adolescent specific evaluations have not made comparisons between different types of adolescent treatment models and have often been found to be methodologically flawed (Drug Strategies, 2002). Importantly, Drug Strategies, a private research institute, recently conducted an exhaustive study that examined the research literature on adolescent treatment. In addition to meta-analysis, the study also included interviews of key individuals involved in adolescent treatment across the United States. Although the review concluded that currently no single treatment model is found to be more effective when compared to others, they did find that effective adolescent treatment requires the inclusion of the family in treatment. The review identified nine key elements critical to the effectiveness of adolescent treatment programs (Drug Strategies, 2002): (a) assessment and treatment matching, (b) comprehensive, integrated treatment approaches, (c) family involvement in treatment, (d) developmentally appropriate programs, (e) engagement and retention in treatment, (f) qualified staff, (g) gender and cultural competence, (h) continuance in post-treatment care, and, (i) treatment evaluation. These elements also serve the additional purpose of providing guidelines to evaluate current treatment programs.

Family-Based Integrative Treatment Models

Prominent among the current integrated models that reflect inclusion of the nine elements for successful adolescent treatment are Multisystemic Therapy (MST; Henggeler et al., 1998), Brief Strategic Family

Therapy (BSFT; Szapocznik et al. 2003), and Multidimensional Family Therapy (MDFT; Liddle, 2004; CSAT, 2004).

Multisystemic Therapy (MST). MST is a family and community-based treatment model that was originally developed in the late 1970s to address the mental health needs of juvenile offenders. Currently, MST is best known for its success in reducing long-term rates of re-arrest and out-of-home placement for violent and chronic juvenile offenders (Henggeler, Schoenwald, Rowland, & Cunningham, 2002). A key feature of MST is its capacity to address the multiple risk factors present in a particular case (hence the name "multisystemic"). Importantly, these risk factors are addressed in a highly individualized and strategic fashion, a careful and ecologically based functional analysis of identified problems (Henggeler et al., 1998). These strategic interventions are selected to provide maximum leverage for achieving a specified goal. Thus, the interventions are comprehensive, but individualized. The development of protective factors is important to the maintenance of therapeutic change. In general, protective factors pertain to the (a) emotional connections in the family, (b) family's connections with a strong indigenous social support network, and (c) development of youth educational and vocational skills and prosocial peer relationships (Henggeler, Clingempeel, Brondino, & Pickrel, 2002).

The Center for Substance Abuse Prevention (CSAP, 2000) has included MST as one of the few treatments of adolescent substance abuse with empirical support. Findings in the first study (Henggeler & Borduin, 1992) showed that MST significantly reduced adolescent reports of a combined index of alcohol and marijuana use at post treatment. The second study (Borduin et al., 1995) reported a 4% reduction in substance-related arrests involving adolescents from the first study. The long term value of MST is documented over a four year period. Family oriented treatment was effective with substance-abusing juvenile offenders (Henggeler, Clingempeel et al., 2002).

Brief Strategic Family Therapy (BSFT). BSFT adapts a structural family systems framework to improve youth's behavior problems by improving family interactions that are presumed to be directly related to the child's symptoms (Szapocznik & Kurtines, 1989; Mitrani, Szapocznik, & Robinson Batista, 2000; Robbins, Mayorga, & Szapocznik, 2003). The target populations in general are children and adolescents between 8 and 17 years of age displaying or at risk for developing behavior problems, including substance abuse. BSFT is a short-term, problem-focused intervention with an emphasis on modifying maladaptive patterns of interactions (Coatsworth, Santisteban, McBride, & Szapocznik, 2001).

The repetitive patterns of family member interactions can be either successful or unsuccessful. BSFT specifically targets the problem-related interaction patterns and establishes a practical plan of intervention to help the family develop more adaptive behaviors (Santisteban et al., 2003).

The BSFT approach consists of four main steps: first, developing a therapeutic alliance with each family member and with the family as a whole; second, identifying family strengths and problem relations that affect the young person's behavior or the ability of parental figures to correct the behavior; third, developing a planful, problem focused, direction-oriented and practical change strategy to capitalize on strengths and to correct problematic family relations (Robbins, Hervis, Mitrani, & Szapocznik, 2001) to increase family competence; and fourth, implementing change strategies and reinforcing family behaviors to sustain new levels of family competence. Strategies include (a) reframing to change the meaning of interactions, changing alliances and shifting interpersonal boundaries (Minuchin, 1974); (b) building conflict resolution skills; and (c) providing parenting guidance and coaching. This approach is recognized as a model program by the Substance Abuse and Mental Health Services Administration (SAMHSA, 2002), and National Institute on Drug Abuse (NIDA, 2002).

Multidimensional Family Therapy (MDFT). MDFT is an outpatient family-based drug abuse treatment for teenage substance abusers (Liddle, 1992; Liddle, 2002a, 2002b). As a developmentally and ecologically oriented treatment, MDFT takes into account the interlocking environmental and individual systems in which clinically referred teenagers reside. Targeted outcomes include reducing the impact of negative factors as well as promoting protective processes in as many areas of the teen's life as possible (Liddle, 1995). Objectives for the adolescent include both transformation of a drug using lifestyle into a developmentally normative lifestyle and improvement in functioning in several developmental domains, including positive peer relations, healthy identity formation, bonding with school and other prosocial institutions, and autonomy within the parent-adolescent relationship. For the parent(s), intermediate objectives include: increased parent commitment and prevention of parental abdication, improved relationship and communication between parent and adolescent, and increased knowledge about parenting practices (e.g., limit-setting, monitoring, appropriate autonomy granting) (Liddle, 2002a). Preliminary results from a randomized trial comparing the clinical effectiveness and relative monetary benefits of MDFT vs. residential treatment for dually diagnosed adolescent substance abusers showed an almost 3:1 differential in the costs of the two treatments favoring MDFT ($384 per week vs. $1,138) (NIDA, 2002; SAMHSA, 2002). Promising results can be obtained by MDFT at a fraction of the cost of residential treatment.

CONCLUSION

The integrated family-based therapies share a number of assumptions in that the adolescent is understood to be embedded within a complex array of interconnected biopsychosocial systems that encompass the individual, family, and extrafamilial (e.g., peer, school, neighborhood, community) factors. The review of risk factors examined multiple levels of risk related to adolescent substance use as represented by individual personality factors, family factors of dysfunction, monitoring, parental addiction, and intrafamilial and extrafamilial deviant peers. The general treatment approaches of the cited family-based therapies focus on accurately assessing the multiple influences and targeting effective intervention strategies designed to support changes throughout a number of systems that affect and serve to reinforce or support the adolescent's problem behaviors. Of additional importance, the models are grounded in a thorough research-based knowledge of key contextual issues in both adolescent and family development (Liddle, 2004). In sum, the integrated family-based models of treatment are representative of some of the most innovative and effective approaches recently developed and currently being implemented in the field (Liddle, 2004).

REFERENCES

Adalbjarnardottir, S., & Hafsteinsson, L. G. (2001). Adolescents' perceived parenting styles and their substance use: Concurrent and longitudinal analyses. *Journal of Research on Adolescence, 11*, 401-423.

American Psychiatric Association (2000). *Diagnostic and statistical manual of mental disorders (4th ed., Text Rev.).* Washington, D.C.: Author.

Andrews, J. A., Hops, H., & Duncan, S. C. (1997). Adolescent modeling of parent substance use: The moderating effect of the relationship with the parent. *Journal of Family Psychology, 11*, 259-270.

Barnow, S., Schuckit, M. A., & Lucht, M. (2002). The importance of a positive family history of alcoholism, parental rejection and emotional warmth, behavioral problems and peer substance use for alcohol problems in teenagers: A path analysis. *Journal of Studies on Alcohol, 63*, 305-312.

Biederman, J., Faraone, S. V., Monuteaux, M. C., & Feighner, J. A. (2000). Patterns of alcohol and drug use in adolescents can be predicted by parental substance use disorders. *Pediatrics, 106*, 792-797.

Bogenschneider, K., Wu, M., & Raffaelli, M. (1998). Parent influences on adolescent peer orientation and substance use: The interface of parenting practices and values. *Child Development, 69*, 1672-1688.

Borduin, C. M., Mann, B. J., Cone, L. T., Henggeler, S. W., Fucci, B. R., Blaske, D. M., et al. (1995). Multisystemic treatment of serious juvenile offenders. Long-term prevention of criminality and violence. *Journal of Consulting and Clinical Psychology, 63*, 569-578.

Bui, K. V. T., Ellickson, P. L., & Bell, R. M. (2000). Cross-lagged relationships among adolescent problem drug use delinquent behavior, and emotional distress. *Journal of Drug Issues, 30*, 283-304.

Center for Substance Abuse Prevention. (2000). *Strengthening America's families: Model family programs for substance abuse and delinquency prevention.* Salt Lake City: Department of Health Promotion and Education, University of Utah.

Center for Substance Abuse Treatment. (2004). *Substance abuse treatment and family therapy.* Treatment Improvement Protocol (TIP) Series, no. 39 (DHHS Publication No. SMA 04-3957). Washington, DC: U.S. Government Printing Office.

Chandy, J. M., Blum, R. W., & Resnick, M. D. (1996). History of sexual abuse and parental alcohol misuse: Risk, outcomes and protective factors in adolescents. *Child and Adolescent Social Work Journal, 13*, 411-432.

Coatsworth, J. D., Santisteban, D. A., McBride, C. K., & Szapocznik, J. (2001). Brief strategic family therapy versus community control: Engagement, retention, and an exploration of the moderating role of adolescent symptom severity. *Family Process, 40*, 313-332.

Coombs, R. H., & Landsverk, J. (1988). Parenting styles and substance use during childhood and adolescence. *Journal of Marriage and the Family, 50*, 473-482.

Curry, L., Fischer, J., Reifman, A., & Harris, K. (2004, March). *Family factors, self-esteem, peer involvement, and adolescent alcohol misuse.* Poster presented at the biennial meeting of the Society for Research on Adolescence, Baltimore., MD.

Dishion, T. J., & McMahon, R. J. (1998). Parental monitoring and the prevention of child and adolescent problem behavior: A conceptual and empirical formulation. *Clinical Child and Family Psychology Review, 1*, 61-75.

Drug Strategies. (2002). *Treating teens: A guide to adolescent drug programs.* Washington: Drug Strategies.

Duncan, T. E., Duncan, S. C., & Hops, H. (1996). The role of parents and older siblings in predicting adolescent substance use: Modeling development via structural equation latent growth methodology. *Journal of Family Psychology, 10*, 158-172.

Ennett, S. T., Bauman, K. E., Foshee, V. A., Pemberton, M., & Hicks, K. A. (2001). Parent-child communication about adolescent tobacco and alcohol use: What do parents say and does it affect youth behavior? *Journal of Marriage and Family, 63*, 48-63.

Farrell, M. P., Barnes, G. M., & Banerjee, S. (1995). Family cohesion as a buffer against the effects of problem-drinking fathers on psychological distress, deviant behavior, and heavy drinking in adolescents. *Journal of Health and Social Behavior, 36*, 377-385.

Fischer, J. L., & Lyness, K. P. (2005). "Families coping with alcohol and substance abuse." In P. S. McKenry & S. J. Price (Eds.), *Families and change: coping with stressful events and transitions (3rd ed.)* (pp. 155-178). Thousand Oaks, CA: Sage.

Fischer, J. L., Pidcock, B. W., Munsch, J., & Forthun, L. (2005). Parental abusive drinking and sibling role differences. *Alcoholism Treatment Quarterly, 23,* 79-97.

Fischer, J. L., & Wampler, R. S. (1994). Abusive drinking in young adults: Personality type and family role as moderators of family-of-origin influences. *Journal of Marriage and the Family, 56,* 469-479.

Foxhall, K. (2001, June). Adolescents aren't getting the help they need. *Monitor on Psychology, 32*(5), 36-42.

Grella, C. E., Joshi, V., & Hser, Y. (2004). Effects of comorbidity on treatment processes and outcomes among adolescents in drug treatment programs. *Journal of Child and Adolescent Substance Abuse, 13*(4), 13-31.

Henggeler, S. W., & Borduin, C. M. (1992). *Mutisystemic therapy adherence scales.* Unpublished instrument, Department of Psychiatry and Behavioral Sciences, Medical University of South Carolina.

Henggeler, S. W., Schoenwald, J. K., Borduin, C. W., Rawland, M. E., & Cunningham, P. B. (1998). *Multisystemic treatment of antisocial behavior in children and adolescents.* New York: Guilford.

Henggeler, S. W., Clingempeel, W. G., Brondino, M. J., & Pickrel, S. G. (2002). Four-year follow-up of multisystemic therapy with substance-abusing and substance-dependent juvenile offenders. *Journal of the American Academy of Child & Adolescent Psychiatry, 41*(7), 868-874.

Henggeler, S. W., Schoenwald, S. K., Rowland, M. D., & Cunningham, P. B. (2002). *Serious emotional disturbance in children and adolescents: Multisystemic therapy.* New York: Guilford Press

Iacono, W. G., Carlson, S. R., Taylor, J., Elkins, I. J., & McGue, M. (1999). Behavioral disinhibition and the development of substance-use disorders: Findings from the Minnesota Twin Study. *Development and Psychopathology, 11,* 869-900.

Jacob, T., & Johnson, S. (1997). Parenting influences on the development of alcohol abuse and dependence. *Alcohol Health and research World, 21,* 204-210.

Jeynes, W. H. (2001). The effects of recent parental divorce on their children's consumption of alcohol. *Journal of Youth and Adolescence, 30,* 305-319.

Johnston, L. D., O'Malley, P. M., Bachman, J. G., & Schulenberg, J. E. (December 19, 2003). *Ecstasy use falls for second year in a row, overall teen drug use drops.* Ann Arbor: University of Michigan News and from http://www.monitoringthefuture.org.

Kafka, R. R., & London, P. (1991). Communication in relationships and adolescent substance use: The influence of parents and friends. *Adolescence, 26,* 587-597.

Kaminer, Y. (2001). Adolescent substance abuse treatment: Where do we go from here? *Psychiatric Services, 52*(2), 147-149.

King, K. M., & Chassin, L. (2004). Mediating and moderated effects of adolescent behavioral undercontrol and parenting in the prediction of drug use disorders in emerging adulthood. *Psychology of Addictive Behaviors, 18,* 239-249.

Liddle, H. A. (1992). Family therapy techniques for adolescents with drug and alcohol problems. In W. Snyder & T. Ooms (Eds.), *Empowering families* (ADAMHA), Monograph from the First National Conference on the Treatment of Adolescent

Drug, Alcohol and Mental Health Problems. Washington, D.C.: United States Public Health Service, U.S. Government Printing Office.

Liddle, H. A. (1995). Conceptual and clinical dimensions of a multidimensional, multisystems engagement strategy in family-based adolescent treatment. *Psychotherapy, 32*, 39-58.

Liddle, H. A. (2002a). Advances in family based therapy for adolescent substance abuse: Findings from the Multidimensional Family Therapy research program. In L.S. Harris (Ed.), Problems of drug dependence 2001: *Proceedings of the 63rd annual scientific meeting* (NIDA Research Monograph No. 182, NIH Publication No. 02-5097, pp. 113-115). Bethesda, MD: National Institute on Drug Abuse.

Liddle, H. A. (2002b). *Multidimensional family therapy for adolescent cannabis users, Cannabis youth treatment (CYT) series, Volume 5.* Center for Substance Abuse Treatment (CSAT), Rockville, MD.

Liddle, H. (2004). Family-based therapies for adolescent alcohol and drug use: Research contributions and future research needs. *Addiction, 99*(2), 76-92.

Luster, T., & Small, S. A. (1997). Sexual abuse history and problems in adolescence: Explaining the effects of moderating variables. *Journal of Marriage and the Family, 59*, 131-142.

Minuchin, S. (1974). *Families and family therapy*. Cambridge, MA: Harvard University Press.

Mitrani, V. B., Szapocznik, J., & Robinson Batista, C. (2000). Structural ecosystems therapy with HIV + African American women. In W. Pequegnat & J. Szapocznik (Eds.), *Working with families in the era of HIV/AIDS* (pp. 243-279). Thousand Oaks, CA: Sage.

National Institute on Alcohol Abuse and Alcoholism (1997). *Youth drinking: Risk factors and consequences* (Alcohol Alert, 37). Retrieved December 20, 2004, from *http://www.niaaa.nih.gov/publications/aa37.htm.*

National Institute on Alcohol Abuse and Alcoholism (2000). *Surgeon General's Report: Alcohol involvement over the life course. In Chapter 1: Drinking over the life span: Issues of biology, behavior, and risk.* Retrieved February 28, 2004, from www.niaaa.gov/publications/10report/chap1.pdf

National Institute on Drug Abuse. (2002). *Monitoring the future: National survey results on drug use, 1975-2001:Volume 1, Secondary school students.* Rockville, MD: NIH.

Pandina, R. J., & Johnson, V. (1990). Serious alcohol and drug problems among adolescents with a family history of alcoholism. *Journal of Studies on Alcohol, 51*, 278-282.

Pidcock, B. W., & Fischer, J. L. (1998). Parental recovery as a moderating variable of adult offspring problematic behaviors. *Alcoholism Treatment Quarterly, 16*, 45-57.

Riggs, P. D. (2003). Treating adolescents for substance abuse and comorbid psychiatric disorders. *Science & Practice Perspectives, 2*, 18-28.

Robbins, M. S., Hervis, O., Mitrani, V. B., & Szapocznik, J. (2001). Assessing changes in family interactions: The structural family systems ratings. In P. K. Kerig & K. M. Lindahl (Eds.), *Family observational coding systems: Resources for systemic research* (pp. 207-224). Mahwah, New Jersey: Erlbaum.

Robbins, M. S., Mayorga, C., & Szapocznik J. (2003). The ecosystemic lense to understanding family functioning. In T. L. Sexton, G. Weeks & M. S. Robbins (Eds.), *Handbook of family therapy* (pp. 21-36). New York: Brunner Routledge.

Santisteban, D. A., Coatsworth, J. D., Perez-Vidal, A., Kurtines, W. M., Schwartz, S. J., LaPerriere, A., et al. (2003). The efficacy of brief strategic family therapy in modifying Hispanic adolescent behavior problems and substance use. *Journal of Family Psychology, 17*(1), 121-135.

Sher, K. J. (1994). Individual-level risk factors. In R. Zucker, G. Boyd & J. Howard (Eds.), *The development of alcohol problems: Exploring the biopsychosocial matrix of risk* (National Institute on Alcohol Abuse and Alcoholism Research Monograph No. 26) (pp. 77–108). Rockville, MD: U.S. Department of Health and Human Services.

Substance Abuse and Mental Health Services Administration. (2002) *Results from the 2001 National Household Survey on Drug Abuse: Volume 1, Summary of national findings.* Rockville, MD: NIH.

Szapocznik, J., & Kurtines, W. M. (1989). *Breakthroughs in family therapy with drug-abusing and problem youth.* New York: Springer.

Szapocznik, J., Hervis, O., & Schwartz, S. (2003). *Brief strategic family therapy for adolescent drug abuse.* (NIH: PUB, no 03-4751). Bethesda, MD: National Institute of Drug Abuse.

VanVoorst, W. A., & Quirk, S. W. (2003). Are relations between parental history of alcohol problems and changes in drinking moderated by positive expectancies? *Alcoholism: Clinical and Experimental Research, 26*, 25-30.

Wampler, R., Fischer, J., Thomas, M., & Lyness, K. (1993). Young adult offspring and their families of origin: Cohesion, adaptability, and addiction. *Journal of Substance Abuse, 5*, 195-201.

Wills, T. A., & Cleary, S. D. (1996). How are social support effects mediated? A test with parental support and adolescent substance use. *Journal of Personality and Social Psychology, 71*, 937-952.

Wills, T. A., & Dishion, T. J. (2004). Temperament and adolescent substance use: A transactional analysis of emerging self-control. *Journal of Clinical and Child and Adolescent Psychology, 33*, 69-81.

Zucker, R., Boyd, G., & Howard, J. (Eds.). (1994). *The development of alcohol problems: Exploring the biopsychosocial matrix of risk* (National Institute on Alcohol Abuse and Alcoholism Research Monograph No. 26). Rockville, MD: U.S. Department of Health and Human Services.

Zuckerman, M., & Kuhlman, D. M. (2000). Personality and risk-taking: Common biosocial factors. *Journal of Personality, 68*, 999-1029.

doi:10.1300/J020v25n01_03

Alcohol Abuse by Older Family Members: A Family Systems Analysis of Assessment and Intervention

Charles D. Stelle, PhD
Jean Pearson Scott, PhD

SUMMARY. The Substance Abuse and Mental Health Services Administration (SAMHSA) describes alcohol related problems with older adults as "underestimated, underidentified, underdiagnosed, and undertreated" (SAMHSA, 2004, p. 1) and describes the phenomenon as an "invisible epidemic" (SAMHSA, 2004, p. 1). The purpose of this review is to address the prevalence and consequences of alcohol abuse in the older adult population by emphasizing the heterogeneity of factors contributing to, and providing a context for, the understanding of alcohol abuse in aging families. Issues surrounding the sensitivity and specificity of assessment of older adult alcohol abusers are covered. Strategies for intervention at both an individual and family level are also included. Although much of the literature available on older adult alcohol use and misuse addresses the consequences, assessment, and intervention from an individualized perspective, this review concludes that a family-oriented approach to intervention may

Charles D. Stelle is affiliated with Bowling Green State University, Department of Human Services, Gerontology Program, 223 Health Center, Bowling Green, OH, 43403-0148 (E-mail: cstelle@bgnet.bgsu.edu).

Jean Pearson Scott is affiliated with the Department of Human Development and Family Studies, Texas Tech University, Lubbock, TX 79409 (E-mail: jean.scott@ttu.edu).

[Haworth co-indexing entry note]: "Alcohol Abuse by Older Family Members: A Family Systems Analysis of Assessment and Intervention." Stelle, Charles D., and Jean Pearson Scott. Co-published simultaneously in *Alcoholism Treatment Quarterly* (The Haworth Press, Inc.) Vol. 25, No. 1/2, 2007, pp. 43-63; and: *Familial Responses to Alcohol Problems* (ed: Judith L. Fischer, Miriam Mulsow, and Alan W. Korinek) The Haworth Press, Inc., 2007, pp. 43-63. Single or multiple copies of this article are available for a fee from The Haworth Document Delivery Service [1-800-HAWORTH, 9:00 a.m. - 5:00 p.m. (EST). E-mail address: docdelivery@haworthpress.com].

Available online at http://atq.haworthpress.com
doi:10.1300/J020v25n01_04

best serve the needs of older alcohol abusers and their support network of family and friends. doi:10.1300/J020v25n01_04 *[Article copies available for a fee from The Haworth Document Delivery Service: 1-800-HAWORTH. E-mail address: <docdelivery@haworthpress.com> Website: <http://www. HaworthPress.com> © 2007 by The Haworth Press, Inc. All rights reserved.]*

KEYWORDS. Alcohol abuse, older adults, assessment, family systems, family therapy

INTRODUCTION

Older individuals drink less and have fewer alcohol related problems than do younger individuals, yet the problems associated with elderly alcohol abuse (EAA) pose significant health challenges, many of which are unique to this age group. Alcohol related problems with older adults have been characterized as "underestimated, underidentified, under-diagnosed, and undertreated" (SAMHSA, 2004, p. 1). A Consensus Panel described substance abuse among older adults as an "invisible epidemic" (SAMHSA, 2004, p. 1). This article examines issues that have perpetuated the invisibility and lack of attention to EAA among older adults, their families, and the professional community.

This review describes the nature of EAA in families. The paper is organized around the concept of the interactive nature of alcohol related behaviors and the aging family system. A description of the nature and magnitude of the problem among older family members is provided. A family systems perspective is then introduced as a theoretical model for understanding the interactive and contextual nature of EAA. With a family systems perspective in mind, the literature on the effects of EAA on older individuals and relationships among the familial system members is discussed. The review of the literature also focuses on the diversity and heterogeneity of EAA. Lastly, assessment of problem drinking and treatment issues among older adults and aging families are discussed.

MAGNITUDE AND DESCRIPTION OF ALCOHOL ABUSE AMONG OLDER ADULTS

The invisibility of EAA is due to multiple factors including ageism, the stigma associated with EAA, lack of awareness of the problematic nature of EAA, clinician beliefs and behaviors, and co-morbidity of EAA

with physical and mental health issues (SAMHSA, 2004). Ageism, in relation to problem drinking and EAA, devalues older adults' quality of life and creates negative perceptions of older individuals in American society. In this way, ageism creates a context where problem behavior and limitations due to EAA are associated with getting older and are therefore not acknowledged or treated. Even when problem drinking is accurately recognized by self or others, a stigma among the current cohort of older adults exists which associates EAA with a personal failing, shame associated with such failure, and the associated reluctance to seek treatment. This stigma pertains not only to older adults themselves, but also to family members, such as partners or adult children, who may be reluctant to assist or refer a family member for treatment. In addition to the stigma associated with EAA, there may be a lack of awareness among family members, especially older family members, of the process and outcomes of EAA.

Of increasing concern is the lack of awareness among clinical staff of EAA. This issue not only deals with recognition of how EAA may present itself differently in an older population, but also that the treatment of EAA is a critical physical and mental health issue. The view that problems in later life are not amenable to treatment often leads to a self-fulfilling prophecy such that treatment options are not considered by family or offered by clinicians. Clinical staff may ignore signs of EAA because they often mimic the symptoms of other common physical and mental conditions. Specifically, EAA is often seen with referrals and diagnoses of mental health problems such as anxiety disorders, depression and dementia. The use of diagnostic instruments with sensitivity, specificity, and appropriateness for older adult populations will assist in the recognition and differential diagnosis of alcohol related problems from comorbid physical and mental health concerns.

Recent demographic changes, and those projected to occur with the continued graying of America, constitute a potential future dilemma of this "invisible epidemic." Health problems associated with problem drinking and the financial costs associated with EAA, will be the most visible signs of the epidemic associated with EAA. U.S. Census projections suggest that the percentage of persons age 65 and over will rise from 12.4 percent in 2000 to 20.7 percent by the year 2050 (U.S. Bureau of Census, 2000). Schonfeld and Dupree (1995), as quoted in SAMHSA (2004), report that "In the United States, it is estimated that 2.5 million older adults have problems related to alcohol, and 21 percent of hospitalized adults over the age of 40 have a diagnosis of alcoholism with related hospital costs as high as $60 billion a year" (Schonfeld & Dupree,

1995, p. 1819). These findings speak to the magnitude of EAA among the current cohort of older adults. In addition, the epidemic nature of alcohol related problems is projected to increase as baby boomers and younger cohorts with more permissive attitudes toward alcohol use than older cohorts continue to age (SAMHSA, 2004). As normal physical changes with aging occur, as well as pathological changes associated with EAA, the health care network and aging families will see an increase in the numbers of alcohol related physical health complications. Lastly, the financial costs of alcohol related problems, both physical and mental, will be borne by family members, federal and state health care and rehabilitation programs (e.g., Medicare, Medicaid). The suggestion of the epidemic nature of EAA is by no means an overstatement.

A FAMILY SYSTEMS PERSPECTIVE ON ALCOHOL ABUSE

Family systems theory provides a number of conceptual tools that help to elucidate the transactional nature of problems associated with EAA. Systems theory describes the linked nature of individual's lives as they exist together and in relation to the external environment (for a general review of systems theory, see Whitchurch & Constantine, 1993; see Westermeyer, 1991 for a review of historical and social contexts). Family systems theory assumes that individuals are members of a holistic, interactive unit. Within this wholeness, there lies an inherent interdependence and mutual influence among members of the family. These assumptions of interrelatedness and interdependence create the necessity of looking beyond individual behavior to describe how the EAA of one family member has an influence on other family members and the family system as a whole. In addition, the patterns and process of interactions among family members are assumed to provide insight into the structure and rules of the system (Day, 1995).

Family systems theory offers guiding assumptions that are particularly relevant to understanding EAA. The recognition that EAA extends in importance and influence beyond the behavior of one individual is the first step in developing recognition of the importance of a family systems perspective on EAA. In his review of alcohol and the family system, Steinglass (1989) suggests that there are five aspects of alcoholism that make a family systems perspective particularly salient. These unique aspects of alcoholism include the chronicity of EAA, that it entails the use of a psychobiologically active drug, that abuse is cyclical

in nature, that it produces predictable behavioral responses, and that it has a definable developmental course (Steinglass, 1989).

Alcoholism, although heterogeneous in nature, is by definition a chronic condition. The importance of using a systems model to understand alcoholism is to examine how the family structure and process are maintained (morphostasis) or adapted (morphogenesis) over the course of time. The depressant effects of alcohol use by the individual presumably impact interactional patterns and dynamics of the family system. In this way, common patterns of interaction, through both verbal and nonverbal communication pathways, will seemingly influence the interdependence of family members and alter the dynamics of their relations as a whole. Alcoholism and EAA tend to be cyclical in nature. Polar states of intoxication and sobriety alter the behavior of individuals in predictable ways. The cycles of intoxication and the resultant predictable behaviors of EAA create "convenient windows" in studying the relationship between alcohol use and family behavior in the alcoholic family (Steinglass, 1989, p. 522). Lastly, alcoholism can be thought of as having a developmental trajectory. Through an individualized pattern of behaviors, alcoholism often demonstrates individual level consistency and a life course of decline. Although there is continued debate on a unitary pattern of alcoholism, types of alcoholism, or varied patterns of alcoholic behaviors, EAA should be conceptualized as a systemic problem within the family that potentially alters the structure and process of family dynamics.

As a result, family involvement in the assessment and intervention of EAA has become more common as the bidirectional influence among members of the family and the family system continue to be explored. For example, the concerns of family members and friends were the most common factor motivating older adults for inpatient treatment for EAA (Finlayson, Hurt, Davis, & Morse, 1988). In this way, we can see that the drinking behaviors of an older family member can cause sufficient problems and concern among family and friends to motivate older adults to seek inpatient treatment. Obtaining help from family members and friends has been shown to lower the likelihood of alcohol-related problems in later-life drinkers (Moos, Schutte, Brennan, & Moos, 2004). Though family can serve to protect against EAA, heavy drinking by significant others (e.g., a husband) has also been discussed as a risk factor for late-onset EAA by women, even under the conditions of spousal loss (Gomberg, 1994). In this way, family members' alcohol abuse may be linked to increasing occurrences of shared drinking behavior, especially with respect to later life.

ALCOHOL USE AND ABUSE BY OLDER
ADULT FAMILY MEMBERS

Prevalence

Identifying the prevalence of problem drinking in later life is complicated by study design, age category, gender, and consumption category. Cross-sectional studies that compare age groups (e.g., Schoenborn & Adams, 2001), but cannot isolate cohort effects, generally find a pattern of lower alcohol use among older age groups compared to younger age groups. The data, categorized by consumption category, show that moderate drinkers are found in similar percentages across all age groups, though percentages of light and heavy drinkers decline in later life. These age differences were similar for men and women though fewer women used alcohol at all ages (Schoenborn & Adams, 2001).

Estimates of EAA vary widely depending on the method used to define EAA (e.g., DSM-IV criteria or other screening methods, National Institute on Alcohol Abuse and Alcoholism (NIAAA) guidelines, definitions of at-risk drinking, heavy drinking, problem-drinking, dependence, drinking in combination with drug use), and the nature of the sample (community dwelling, hospitalized, nursing home, geographic location). Consequently, estimates vary widely and may be confusing and even contradictory. The 1988 National Health Interview Survey, using more stringent DSM-III criteria, yielded a one-year prevalence rate of 1.4% among those persons age 65 and older compared to a one-year prevalence rate of 8.6% for the national sample as a whole.

Prevalence rates from other community studies ranged from 2 to 22% (Dufour & Fuller, 1995). Studies using hospitalized samples documented that older persons with drinking problems were overrepresented (10% or more of persons age 65 and over) (Dufour & Fuller, 1995). Similarly, case management records of 1668 clients of a community based mental health center established that 9.6% of their self-referred and gatekeeper initiated older adult clientele were diagnosed with primary or secondary EAA (Jinks & Raschko, 1990). Lifetime EAA and dependence were high (49%) in a sample of Veterans Affairs (VA) nursing home residents (18% active, 31% inactive) and 50% of those who were active drinkers remained so at a three year follow-up (Joseph, Ganzini, & Atkinson, 1995; Joseph, Rasmussen, Ganzini, & Atkinson, 1997). Another review of epidemiological studies found prevalence rates from 2 to 45% for EAA (Johnson, 2000). These studies demonstrate the wide variation in reported rates of EAA due to the type of samples and the criteria for diagnosis.

There are few longitudinal studies of alcohol consumption and abuse, and the studies that do exist are contradictory. Fillmore (1988) and Fillmore et al.'s (1991) meta-analyses of longitudinal studies found age declines in general alcohol consumption and, when broken out by consumption level, declines with both heavy and problem drinking, but not with moderate drinking. Moos et al. (2004) examined late middle aged drinkers over a 10 year span to investigate drinking change over time. Measurements of alcohol use and abuse from baseline, one year, four year, and 10 year increments showed that the proportion of individuals who consumed alcohol declined (Moos et al., 2004). In addition, women and men showed similar declines in usage and comparable rates of drinking problems (Moos et al., 2004). Studies that have isolated cohort, period, and age effects have yielded inconsistent results. Data from the Normative Aging Study were used in a comparison at two observation points where cohort effects were found to be largely responsible for lower rates of drinking for the older cohorts across time (Glynn, Bouchard, LoCastro, & Laird, 1985). Chaikelson, Arbuckle, Lapidus., and Gold (1994) studied trajectories of change in alcohol consumption of 70 World War II veterans and found a pattern of change in which drinking increased from young adulthood to middle age, leveled off, and then decreased sharply in the participants' 70s and 80s. In a Dutch study, the increase in alcohol consumption over 30 years in all five 10 year cohorts was attributed to period effects, i.e., more liberal attitudes toward drinking (Neve, Diederiks, Knibbe, & Drop, 1993). Aldwin, Levenson, and Gilmer (2004) cite their 1998 study (Levenson, Aldwin, & Spiro, 1998) as the first sequential study that statistically tested the differential effects of age, cohort, and period on alcohol consumption. They followed cohorts over an 18 year period and concluded that consumption in adulthood was largely a function of period effects. Drinking increased for all ages during the 1970s and declined in the 1980s. Age had a minor effect as not as many older adults drank, but those who did, did not lower their drinking appreciably (Aldwin et al., 2004). These findings suggest that age, period, and cohort may be in operation in the drinking behavior of older adults.

Underdiagnosis

Older adults are less likely to receive a diagnosis of alcoholism when compared to younger adults with the same presenting complaints and behaviors (Booth, Blow, Cook, Bunn, & Fortney, 1992). Alcoholism may not be recognized because older problem drinkers often present with major physical and/or mental health problems with symptoms that mask a drinking problem. Specifically, EAA may mimic the symptoms of depression, dementia, stroke, cardiac problems, malnutrition, falls and accidents, and prescription and over-the-counter drug reactions. Furthermore, health care providers may be reluctant to screen for alcoholism in order to avoid embarrassment to older patients and their families. Health care professionals may use screening criteria that are inappropriate for older persons, not realizing that physiological changes with age make the body less tolerant of alcohol in later life.

Consequences of Alcohol Abuse

The health consequences of EAA and biochemistry of alcohol metabolism in older adults have been well-documented over time (for a review, see Beresford & Gomberg, 1995; Stoddard & Thompson, 1996). Active EAA in a Veterans Administration (VA) health care setting was also linked to younger ages at death, even when compared to individuals with a history of EAA (Joseph et al., 1997). Although some of these deaths were related to EAA, such as liver disease, increased mortality was also linked to smoking related disease (e.g., chronic obstructive pulmonary disease) and other causes of death (e.g., heart disease).

In a review of the literature on alcohol and the older adult population, Stoddard and Thompson (1996) suggest that cues to EAA include falls, cognitive dysfunction, sexual dysfunction, incontinence, malnutrition, tremors, weight loss/poor appetite, self-neglect, tobacco dependency, and complications related to concurrent drug use. Older men who had a history of alcoholism concomitant with depression had more difficulty with chronic illness compared to those diagnosed with major depression with no history of EAA (Cook, Winokur, Garvey, & Beach, 1991). In a study of 216 older adult inpatients, Finlayson et al. (1988) found that tobacco dependence (67%), organic brain syndrome (25%), atypical or mixed organic brain disorder (19%) and affective disorder (19%) were the most common psychiatric conditions associated with later-life alcoholics. Major depressive disorders have also been found to be associated with EAA. In a historical prospective study of 58 men over the age of 55 with a history of non-bipolar depression, almost 28% were found to have a history of alcoholism (Cook et al., 1991). Although there are similarities found in the impact of alcohol abuse, there is considerable variability in identifying individuals who are more or less likely to abuse alcohol in later life. These multiple co-morbidities create challenges for prompt, accurate diagnosis of EAA and often result in underdiagnosis.

Heterogeneity of Alcohol Abuse in Older Adults

Reports on the prevalence of EAA vary widely. Issues such as the reasons for abuse, the onset of EAA, gender, culture, and location can influence the etiology, duration, and prevalence of abuse. In a study of alcoholism in older adult inpatients, Finlayson et al. (1988) found that late-onset alcoholics reported a higher frequency of stressor events (e.g., physical health problems) when compared to early-onset alcoholics. Schonfeld and Dupree (1990) suggest that older adults with alcohol problems are often also found to drink in response to loneliness, reduced or poor social support networks, and psychological issues such as depression and/or anxiety. In addition to potential reactive drinking, a family history of alcoholism can lead to higher prevalence of lifetime drinking when compared to predictors such as age, race, and gender (Grant, 1998). As such, age at onset of drinking and a family history of alcohol abuse can be seen as an indicator of genetic factors, shared environmental factors, or a combination of the two as reasons contributing to EAA.

In terms of the potential course of EAA, one of the major issues of heterogeneity is the timing of EAA as early or late-onset. Early-onset EAA may be envisioned as a lifelong pattern of problem behavior originating in earlier years or as a late-onset problem with heavy drinking beginning in later life. In his review of the literature, Atkinson (1994) suggests that 1/4 to 2/3 of aging alcoholics have an initial onset of problem drinking after the age of 60. Risk factors for late-onset alcoholism include the timing of exposure to alcohol, demographic factors, psychiatric comorbidity, family alcoholism, and life stress (Atkinson, 1994). There may also be psychiatric co-morbidity associated with problem drinking, however; no differences were found between early-onset and late-onset abusers among inpatients being treated for alcoholism (Finlayson et al., 1988). Family alcoholism tends to be a less important factor in late-onset cases of EAA than in early-onset drinking (Atkinson, Tolson, & Turner, 1990). Life stress has also been mentioned as an indicator for late-onset problem drinking. Finlayson et al. (1988) noted that the number of life stressors, such as retirement or physical health problems, were about twice as likely in the late-onset alcoholic group when compared to the early-onset alcoholic inpatients. Similarly, a study of a community sample by Moos, Brennan, and Moos (1991) found that life stressors such as health problems or financial difficulties were associated with EAA. From these studies, two different profiles emerge based on the age of onset of alcohol abuse. Late-onset alcohol abuse appears to be associated with the inability to cope with stressful life course events that are associated with contextual factors rather than genetic predispositions that are more characteristic of early-onset drinkers.

Gender differences are reflected in the rates and etiology of EAA. Men are often found to have higher rates of EAA when compared to women (Jinks & Raschko, 1990). In a study of 161 individuals assessed by Elderly Services of Spokane to have primary or secondary EAA, 70% and 63% respectively were male. Of the secondary diagnoses of EAA, concurrent dementia and moderate depression were the most common primary diagnoses. In a cross-cultural study of gender differences in EAA, the general rates of alcohol use and abuse were found to be influenced by gender. Men had longer lifetime drinking patterns and women were more likely to be lifetime abstainers (Wilsnack, Vogeltanz, Wilsnack, & Harris, 2000). In addition, men and women's drinking patterns across multiple cultural groups declined across increasing age in cross-sectional age comparisons. However, although men and women were found to have similar general consumption rates, heavy drinking was still more likely to be associated with men. There may also be gender differences in the development and course of EAA in men and women. Older men were more likely to be married, divorced, or separated and have a longer history of EAA, although women were more likely to be widowed and have a more recent onset of EAA (Gomberg, 1995). The abuse of alcohol by women may also be underdiagnosed by physicians. Joseph et al. (1995) suggest that studies utilizing interviews, as compared to clinical diagnosis, would be more likely to accurately assess the prevalence of EAA in women in a nursing home population. For example, Curtis, Geller, Stokes, Levine, and Moore (1989) found no instance of diagnosis by physicians for white, female patients over the age of 60. This compares to 9 male participants who were positively screened for alcoholism. The authors conclude that the stereotype of an elderly individual with alcoholism continues to be associated with gender with males having higher rates of EAA.

There is a paucity of research investigating potential differences in the prevalence of EAA in terms of ethnic or cultural differences. In a study of admissions into the Johns Hopkins Hospital, Curtis et al. (1989) found 21% of patients over the age of 60 were positively screened for alcoholism. Of these patients, elderly patients with alcoholism were significantly more likely to be African-American. Latino elderly have a higher incidence of health conditions such as diabetes and liver disease, that are brought on or exacerbated by drinking and EAA (Gelfand, 2003). A legacy of near annihilation, forced assimilation, and lifelong discrimination are influential factors in the higher prevalence of problem drinking and alcohol abuse among Native Americans. The sixth leading cause of death among Native Americans is chronic liver disease and cirrhosis; a rate higher than that found in the general population (Anderson, 2001). Native American elderly have higher rates of chronic diseases compared to Anglo elderly that are exacerbated with drinking such as diabetes, liver, and kidney disease (Gelfand, 2003). These findings, though limited, document the serious consequences of EAA among minority populations, especially Native Americans. At a cross-cultural level, Wilsnack et al. (2000) found that rates of alcohol consumption were similar across multiple cultural groups. Rates of abstention and consumption across groups (including Australian, Canadian, Czech, Finnish, Dutch, Swedish, and American) demonstrated cross-sectional findings of increasing likelihood of abstention and reduced consumption with age categories.

An additional issue of heterogeneity is the location and setting of EAA. Nursing home populations, though only representing approximately 5% of the older adult population at any time, have received significant attention. In a meta-analysis of alcohol and drug use and abuse in nursing homes, Joseph et al. (1995) found that prevalence rates of alcohol use associated problems are found in the range of 2.8 to 49% of the population depending on the settings and methods utilized. Their conclusions regarding issues of heterogeneity suggest that prevalence rates of EAA depend on time frame (e.g., lifetime alcohol use vs current diagnosis) and characteristics of the setting (e.g., facility characteristics; higher rates of younger, male populations; or Veteran Affairs facilities).

Individual Assessment of Alcohol Abuse in Older Adults

There are a multitude of ways that screening and diagnosis for EAA and alcoholism can take place that vary according to study, location, and approach. Issues of diagnosis in the literature are further complicated by the use of overlapping classification systems using terminology such as alcohol abuse, misuse, dependence, heavy drinking, alcoholism, and varying levels of substance abuse disorders (Dehart & Hoffman, 1995). In addition to confusing and overlapping terminology, issues of the comorbidity of EAA with psychiatric conditions make assessment and diagnosis more complex and challenging (Dehart & Hoffman, 1995).

Screening for EAA in the adult population, as a mechanism of prevention, is complicated by the sensitivity (true positives) and specificity (avoiding false negatives) of available measures (DeHart & Hoffman, 1995). Screening assessment measures commonly used for EAA and dependence are often assumed to be valid for older adult populations based on their validity in younger populations. Although structured interviews using DSM-IV criteria can be employed to assess EAA problems, the most commonly used screening includes some type of written assessment. Dehart and Hoffman (1995) reviewed the literature on common assessments of alcohol abuse and concluded that new measures need to be evaluated and validated in order to more accurately identify EAA.

In another review, O'Connell et al. (2004) evaluated screening instruments for the detection of alcohol use disorders in older adult populations. The CAGE (derived from the four questions assessing alcohol use through question on Cut down of drinking, Annoyed by others regarding drinking, Guilt about drinking, using alcohol as an Eye-Opener) was the most widely used screening instrument. The CAGE was followed by the Michigan Alcohol Screening Test (MAST), the Alcohol Use Disorders identification Test (AUDIT), and variations on the AUDIT in terms of frequency of use. The sensitivity and specificity of the instruments were found to vary widely depending on the prevalence and type of EAA being studied and the clinical characteristics of the population (O'Connell et al., 2004). The authors conclude that the selection of a screening instrument must be done with issues such as ease of use, patient acceptability, sensitivity and specificity of the instrument, and the population characteristics taken into account (O'Connell et al., 2004).

The discrepancy between structured interviews and screening instruments can be problematic. Dehart and Hoffman (1995) suggest that instruments such as the CAGE and MAST may not be equally valid for screening of all older adults considering the instruments were normed on a male population. In a CAGE reliability meta-analysis, Shields and Carusso (2004) found an association between increasing age and CAGE score, but the sample age ranged from 17.4 to 44.9 years of age. Using the CAGE questionnaire and Short Michigan Alcohol Screening Test, Curtis et al. (1989) found that 60% of younger patients, aged 60 and younger, were identified both by questionnaire and physicians as alcoholics. By contrast, only 37% of older patients (age 60 +) were correctly identified by both the survey instruments and physician diagnosis.

The discussion of underdiagnosis and underutilization of EAA programs underscores the need to correctly identify and intervene into the lives of older adults who abuse alcohol. Even when correctly identified as alcoholics, older adults (60 +) were significantly less likely to have treatment recommended. In addition, even if treatment was recommended, it was less likely to be initiated by physicians in the older age group compared to the younger (age 60 or younger) group (Curtis et al., 1989).

Individual Intervention

Issues of intervention depend upon the theoretical orientation to EAA as an acute or chronic condition (Dehart & Hoffman, 1995). An orientation to alcohol dependence as an acute condition often translates to limited intervention and health care policies that inappropriately view EAA as episodic. Alternatively, EAA may be seen as a condition that involves recovery, remission, management, and potential aggravation. In addition, the recognition of EAA subtypes may also aid in intervention. For example, Atkinson (1990) suggests that abusers be classified as early-onset (before age 40), midlife-onset (aged 41-59), and later-life onset (age 60 +) to aid in understanding the etiology and course of EAA.

The data on intervention for EAA highlight the potential effectiveness of brief interventions. In a controlled clinical trial of younger and older alcohol abusers, Lemke and Moos (2002) found that younger and older inpatient participants showed similar outcomes, prognosis, and response to treatment orientation. Older adult participants were in poorer physical health and had lower cognitive status, however, they were also drinking less, had fewer drinking-related problems, fewer psychological symptoms, more social support, more adaptive coping, and fewer barriers to abstinence. Similarly, Fleming, Manwell, Barry, Adams, and Stauffacher (1999) conducted a controlled clinical trial of 158 older adults to test the efficacy of brief physician interventions. These interventions consisted of 2 face-to-face education sessions (the first intervention and a reinforcement session) focusing on health behaviors, alcohol abuse education, and the adverse effects of alcohol use. In addition, contracting occurred between the participants in the intervention group and physicians to reduce the patient's alcohol use. Also included were phone follow-ups between clinic nurses and participants after each visit. The results comparing the intervention group to matched controls demonstrate a 34% reduction in 7-day alcohol use, a 74% reduction in mean number of binge drinking episodes, and a 62% reduction in the percentage of older adults drinking more that 21 drinks per week.

Although many individual intervention strategies (such as psycho-dynamic, Twelve Step, social support, behavioral, and cognitive-behavioral) have been employed, Schonfeld and Dupree (1995) conclude that only those involving behavioral intervention have demonstrated treatment effectiveness in older adults. These behavioral approaches included those that utilize basic behavioral concepts (e.g., conditioning) and those that extend to covert behaviors through self-management and cognitive-behavioral principles (e.g., relapse prevention). In addition, the authors' review suggests that age-specific treatment options produce better outcomes than when mixed treatment of younger and older alcoholics are utilized. The authors suggest that age-specific group treatment, whereby groups are limited to older alcohol abusers, allows for focus on EAA issues such as overcoming depression, loneliness, and rebuilding social support networks (Schonfeld and Dupree, 1995) that are more likely in EAA.

Individual level treatment of older alcohol abusers must also take into account limited personal resources and benefits to pay for services, caregivers with limited knowledge of aging, longer detoxification time, and the need for physical accommodation of disability and health limitations (Stoddard & Thompson, 1996). When examining outcomes of individual level treatment, Lemke and Moos (2002) found that initial status of incoming older adult inpatients (specifically older men in a VA mixed age alcohol treatment program) was the strongest predictor of discharge functioning. Specifically, older men with higher cognitive functioning (measured by abstraction skill using the Shipley Institute of Living Scale), stronger motivation for treatment (from the Determination and Action subscales of the Stages of Change Readiness and Treatment Eagerness Scale), and higher levels of social support (from the Life Stressors and Social Resources Inventory) showed marked improvement. Older men, as compared to their middle-age and younger counterparts, scored significantly lower on cognitive functioning and motivation for treatment, but higher in levels of received social support and social engagement. In terms of treatment efficacy, older men with higher levels of abstract reasoning skill, more motivation for change, and increased social support resources showed the most improvement. The nature of the study, in terms of a naturalistic cross-sectional investigation, limits the ability to draw conclusions on the efficacy of specific treatments received or whether older men would have benefited differentially with age-specific treatment. Nevertheless, the study does point to the importance of incoming status for treatment efficacy and the distinctiveness of EAA inpatient participants.

Family Level Intervention

Family systems theory emphasizes the dynamic and interactive nature of the structure and process of family relationships. In the discussion of family-involved approaches to the treatment of alcoholism, Chan (2003) points to the need to view the family as a unit that is reciprocally deterministic and seeks to maintain stability in the face of disturbances in the family through interaction and communication patterns. With respect to EAA, there is a need to recognize the bidirectional influence between the abusing individual and the family system. In this way, the older individual has an effect upon, and is influenced by, the other members of the family system. Further, the attempt to maintain homeostasis within this system can be seen in the use of defense mechanisms, such as denial of alcohol associated problems, and the maintenance of stability and avoidance of change.

Within a family systems framework, concern expressed by family members and friends regarding older adult's drinking can have an influence on the likelihood of seeking treatment and also differs according to demographic characteristics of the abuser (Room, Matzger, & Weisner, 2004). Pressure can be placed on an older adult by spouses, family members, and friends to seek intervention for EAA. After controlling for severity, individuals with higher degrees of dependence and increased social consequences related to their drinking behavior were most likely to receive pressure from all sources. At a demographic level, individuals with higher incomes were more likely to have pressure placed by a spouse, although those with lower incomes were more likely to receive pressure from siblings, other family members, and friends. Older individuals were more likely to be pressured for treatment of EAA by adult children (Room et al., 2004).

Intervention into the family system can also serve a viable role in intervention for adults exhibiting issues of EAA. Vetere and Henley (2001) introduce a process of integrating systemic psychotherapy into group analytic psychotherapy for intervention into couples and families experiencing EAA. By incorporating Prochaska and DiClemente's (1992) model of change, the authors propose that intervention can be employed at any stage of the spiraling movement that individuals engage in as they progress through recovery by means of precontemplation, contemplation, preparation, action and maintenance.

There is also a need to see the heterogeneity of EAA as an indicator of the necessity to correspond treatment with subtypes of EAA (Beutler et al., 1993). Beutler et al. suggested that there are internalizing and externalizing types of alcoholics based on a review of treatment efficacy, patient coping style, drinking patterns, and family dynamics. Internalizing alcoholics are those individuals whose drinking patterns are stable over time and interwoven with family interactions. Externalizing alcoholics, on the other hand, are characterized by episodic drinking, interpersonal disturbances, and behaviors which are impulsive and aggressive. This subtype may benefit more from cognitive-behavioral treatments than from family-involved intervention (Beutler et al., 1993). For those individuals who seek couple or family-involved therapy, it is suggested that treatment revolve around therapists aligning with the couple/family against the external threat of alcohol.

In a demonstration project on the treatment modalities useful for elderly alcoholics, Dunlop, Skorney, and Hamilton (1982) describe a range of treatment options including intervention, aftercare, couple's counseling, and family-involved group treatment. Dunlop et al. (1982) discuss some of the characteristics unique to the group process with an older adult population including issues such as disability/impairment accommodation, jargon usage, potential cohort limitations on self-disclosure, and the need for same-age peers in group treatment. The focus of intervention on the strengths of the individual, and the strength of the family context, can be highly adaptive as it takes advantage of the adaptive abilities of the individual to cope that have been developed over a lifetime (Perkins & Tice, 1999). In a meta-analysis of family-involved therapy for alcoholism across age groups, Edwards and Steinglass (1995) conclude that family-involved therapy is marginally more effective than individual treatment. The effectiveness of treatment is mediated by gender, investment in relationships, and perceived support for abstinence from a spouse (Edwards & Steinglass, 1995).

The issue of codependency helps to underscore the potential need to view EAA within a dynamic systems approach. Scaturo, Hayes, Sagula, and Walter (2000) argue that EAA and codependency are theoretically linked to family system concepts. Therapeutic considerations in assessing and treating EAA in families involve confronting codependent behavior, psychoeducational intervention, and self-exploration. The confrontation of codependency involves addressing and validating the well-intentioned codependent individual although assisting the codependent individual in finding new ways of being useful within their role in the family system. Psychoeducational intervention targets the misattribution of behavior as codependent and helps to assure that family members do not become overly-critical of their role in the use of alcohol by an older family member. Lastly, self-exploration provides for emotional growth of the codependent family member although avoiding overly-critical self attributions. These mechanisms of intervention at the family level assist in the creation of a supportive environment for the treatment of the older family member abusing alcohol.

In addition to family level intervention, Holder (2001) details the need to view EAA as a community level problem. Community level intervention recognizes that EAA is part of a community life and that the community level must be considered within an accurate systems perspective. As such, community planners and policy makers need to consider how their particular community influences rates of EAA and possibly contributes to EAA. Holder (2001) argues that alcohol prevention strategies will often need to be different, and consequently require a different perspective, than more broadly based state and national programs. In addition, alcohol misuse and abuse is not limited to an individual or an event, but has emergent rippling consequences on the community. These effects include issues such as disrupted families, lost economic production at the familial and community levels, and higher costs for medical care. As such, a systems perspective on EAA needs to view alcohol problems as products of dynamic relationships between older adults, family members, and the community, rather than the difficulty of one individual. Holder (2001) suggests that alcohol treatment at the community level must adequately balance a program's scientific evidence of potential efficacy with cost-effectiveness to sufficiently address alcohol prevention in the twenty-first century.

It is important to note that there are problems associated with family-involved approaches to treatment of alcohol abuse regardless of the age group concerned (Chan, 2003). To date, there is no agreed-upon family therapy orientation to the treatment of alcoholism. The use of labels within a family-involved treatment approach (e.g., lost child, scapegoat) may also lead to unnecessary negative self descriptions. Family-involved therapies must also address the micro level issues of the individual and not neglect intrapersonal reasons and effects of EAA while focusing on the family unit. In addition, many of the approaches to alcohol treatment, even those used with a family-involved approach, remain behavioristic in orientation and fail to address the holistic nature and circular causality of family systems (Chan, 2003). Lastly, a family-involved approach is not necessarily a systems focus as it may fail to deal with macro level issues such as public policy, societal attitudes, or the multiple environments (e.g., nursing home, assisted living, community residing) that influence where EAA takes place. In addition, there may be unrecognized barriers or attitudes of older family members to family-involved intervention. For example, Lemke and Moos (2002) found that although older participants had positive views of multiple intervention programs, they utilized less family therapy when compared to younger participants. These difficulties exist as weakness to the current use of family-involved approaches to EAA, rather than direct criticism of the utility of family-involved approaches. As research into the use of a family systems perspective on EAA and family-involved treatment programs with older adults continues, the conditions under which it is more effective and desirable will be explicated.

CONCLUSION

Alcohol abuse within the older adult population is becoming a recognized problem and will be recognized even more so as the population continues to age. Although prevalence rates depend on many factors, the "invisible epidemic" of EAA continues. Underdiagnosis, differential diagnosis, accurate assessment, and intervention consensus continue to be problematic. At the individual level, issues such as the heterogeneity of risk factors, assessment, and intervention have been investigated. However, the connection between individual EAA and family and community process is less well-documented. There is a growing, but inconsistent, body of literature that indicates the need to view EAA within a family systems perspective. For example, Edwards and Steinglass (1995) conclude that family-involved therapy is more effective than individual treatment while Schonfeld and Dupree (1995) conclude that only those interventions involving behavioral strategies have demonstrated treatment effectiveness in older adults. An additional area for investigation remains the question of group setting. Schonfeld and Dupree (1995) suggest that age-specific treatment options produce better outcomes while evidence also exists for the efficacy of mixed-age treatments (Lemke & Moos, 2002). These questions remain to be fully addressed, but the need for EAA to be recognized and to receive effective intervention continues.

REFERENCES

Aldwin, C. M., Levenson, M. R., & Gilmer, D. F. (2004). The interface between physical and mental health. In C. M. Aldwin & D. F. Gilmer (Eds.), *Health, illness, and optimal aging: Biological and psychosocial perspectives* (pp. 229-253). Thousand Oaks, CA: Sage.

Anderson, R. (2001) National vital statistics reports. Deaths: Leading causes for 1999. Retrieved April 15, 2002, from http://www.cdc.gov/nchs/data/nvsr49/nvsr49_11.pdf

Atkinson, R. (1990). Aging and alcohol use disorders: Diagnostic issues in the elderly. *International Psychogeriatrics, 2*(1), 55-72.

Atkinson, R. (1994). Late onset problem drinking in older adults. *International Journal of Geriatric Psychiatry, 9*, 321-326.

Atkinson, R., Tolson, R., & Turner, J. (1990). Later versus early onset problem drinking in older men. *Alcoholism: Clinical and Experimental Research, 14*, 574-579.

Beresford, T., & Gomborg, E. (Eds.) (1995). *Alcohol and aging.* New York: Oxford University.

Beutler, L., Patterson, K., Jacob, T., Shoham, V., Yost, E., & Rohrbach, M. (1993). Matching treatment to alcoholism subtypes. *Psychotherapy: Theory, Research, Practice, Training, 30*(3), 463-472.

Booth, B. M., Blow, F. C., Cook, C. A., Bunn, J. Y. & Fortney, J. C. (1992). Age and ethnicity among hospitalized alcoholics: A nationwide study. *Alcoholism: Clinical and Experimental Research, 16*, 435-442.

Chaikelson, J. S., Arbuckle, T. Y., Lapidus, S., & Gold, D. P. (1994). Measurement of life-time alcohol consumption. *Journal of Studies on Alcohol, 55*, 133-140.

Chan, J. (2003). An examination of family-involved approaches to alcoholism treatment. *The Family Journal: Counseling and Therapy for Couples and Families, 11*(2), 129-138.

Cook, B., Winokur, G., Garvey, M., & Beach, V. (1991). Depression and previous alcoholism in the elderly. *British Journal of Psychiatry, 158*, 72-75.

Curtis, R., Geller, G., Stokes, E., Levine, D., & Moore, R. (1989). Characteristics, diagnosis, and treatment of alcoholism in elderly patients. *Journal of the American Geriatrics Society, 37*, 310-316.

Day, R. (1995). Family systems theory. In R. Day, K. Gilbert, B. Settles & W. Day (Eds.), *Research and theory in family science* (pp. 91-101). Pacific Grove, CA: Brooks/Cole.

Dehart, S., & Hoffman, N. (1995). Screening and diagnosis of "alcohol abuse and dependence" in older adults. *The International Journal of the Addictions, 30*(13-14), 1717-1747.

Dufour, M., & Fuller, R. (1995). Alcohol in the elderly. *Annual Review of Medicine, 46*, 123-132.

Dunlop, J., Skorney, B., & Hamilton, J. (1982). Group treatment for elderly alcoholics and their families. *Social Work with Groups, 5*(1), 87-92.

Edwards, M., & Steinglass, P. (1995). Family therapy treatment outcomes for alcoholism, *Journal of Marital and Family Therapy, 21*(4), 475-509.

Fillmore, K. M. (1988). *Alcohol use across the life course: A critical review of 70 years of international longitudinal research.* Toronto: Addiction Research Foundation.

Fillmore, K. M., Harka, E., Johnstone, B. M., Leino, E. V., Motoyoshi, M., & Temple, M. T. (1991). The collaborative alcohol-related longitudinal project. *British Journal of Addiction, 86*, 1221-1268.

Finlayson, R., Hurt, R., Davis, L., & Morse, R. (1988). Alcoholism in elderly persons: A study of the psychiatric and psychosocial features of 216 inpatients. *Mayo Clinic Proceedings, 63*, 761-768.

Fleming, M., Manwell, L., Barry, K., Adams, W., & Stauffacher, E. (1999). Brief physician intervention for alcohol problems in older adults: A randomized community based trial. *Journal of Family Practice, 48*(5), 378-384.

Glynn, R. J., Bouchard, G. R., LoCastro, J. S., & Laird, N. M. (1985). Aging and generational effects on drinking behaviors in men: Results from the Normative Aging Study. *American Journal of Public Health, 75*, 1413-1419.

Gelfand, D. (2003). *Aging and ethnicity: Knowledge and services (2nd ed.).* New York: Springer.

Gomberg, E. (1994). Risk factors for drinking over a women's life span. *Alcohol Health and Research World, 18*(3), 220-227.

Gomberg, E. (1995). Older women and alcohol: Use and abuse. In M. Galanter (Ed.), *Recent developments in alcoholism: Vol. 12, Alcoholism and women* (pp. 61-79). New York: Plenum.

Grant, B. (1998). The impact of a family history of alcoholism on the relationship between age at onset of alcohol use and DSM-IV alcohol dependence. *Alcohol Health and Research World, 22*(2), 144-147.

Holder, H. (2001). Prevention of alcohol problems in the 21st century: Challenges and opportunities. *The American Journal on Addictions, 10*, 1-15.

Jinks, M., & Raschko, R. (1990). A profile of alcohol and prescription drug abuse in a high-risk community based elderly population. *The Annals of Pharmacotherapy, 24*, 971-975.

Johnson, I. (2000). Alcohol problems in old age: A review of recent epidemiological research. *International Journal of Geriatric Psychiatry, 15*, 575-581.

Joseph, C. L., Ganzini, L., & Atkinson, R. (1995). Screening for alcohol use disorders in the nursing home. *Journal of the American Geriatrics Society, 43*, 368-373.

Joseph, C., Rasmussen, J., Ganzini, L., & Atkinson, R. (1997). Outcome of nursing home care for residents with alcohol use disorders. *International Journal of Geriatric Psychiatry, 12*, 767-772.

Lemke, S., & Moos, R. (2002). Prognosis of older patients in mixed-age alcoholism treatment programs. *Journal of Substance Abuse Treatment, 22*(1), 33-43.

Levenson, M. R., Aldwin, C. M., & Spiro, A. III. (1998). Age, cohort, and period effects on alcohol consumption and problem drinking: Findings from the Normative Aging Study. *Journal of Studies on Alcohol, 59*, 712-722.

Moos, R., Brennan, P., & Moos, B. (1991). Short-term processes of remission and nonremission among late-life problem drinkers. *Alcoholism: Clinical and Experimental Research, 15*, 948-955.

Moos, R., Schutte, K., Brennan, P., & Moos, B. (2004). Ten-year patterns of alcohol consumption and drinking problems among older women and men. *Addiction, 99*, 829-838.

Neve, R., Diederiks, J., Knibbe, R., & Drop, M. (1993) Developments in drinking behavior in the Netherlands from 1958 to 1989, a cohort analysis. *Addiction, 88*(5), 611-621.

O'Connell, H., Chin, A., Hamilton, F., Cunningham, C., Walsh, J., Coakley, D., & Lawlor, B. (2004). A systematic review of the utility of self-report alcohol screening instruments in the elderly. *International Journal of Geriatric Psychiatry, 19*(11), 1074-1166.

Perkins, K., & Tice, C. (1999). Family treatment of older adults who misuse alcohol: A strengths perspective. *Journal of Gerontological Social Work, 31*(4), 169-185.

Prochaska, J., & DiClemente, C. (1992). Stages of change in the modification of problem behaviors. In M. Herson, R. Eisler, R., & P. Miller (Eds.), *Progress in behavior*. Sycamore, NJ: Sycamore.

Room, R., Matzger, H., & Wesiner, C. (2004). Sources of informal pressure on problematic drinkers to cut down or seek treatment. *Journal of Substance Abuse, 9*(6), 280-295.

Scaturo, D., Hayes, T., Sagula, D., & Walter, T. (2000). The concept of codependency and its context within family systems theory. *Family Therapy, 27*(2), 63-70.

Schoenborn, C. A., & Adams, P. F. (2001). Alcohol use among adults: United States 1997-1998. *Advanced Data From Vital and Health Statistics*, #324, whole issue.

Schonfeld, L., & Dupree, L. (1990). Older problem drinkers-long term and late-life onset abusers: What triggers their drinking? *Aging, 361*, 5-8.

Schonfeld, L., & Dupree, L. (1995). Treatment approaches for older problem drinkers. *International Journal of the Addictions, 30*(13 & 14), 1819-1842.

Shields, A., & Caruso, J. (2004). A reliability induction and reliability generalization study of the CAGE questionnaire. *Educational and Psychological Measurement, 64*(2), 254-270.

Steinglass, P. (1989). Alcohol and the family system. In C. Ramsey Jr. (Ed.), *Family systems in medicine* (pp. 519-535). New York, NY: Guilford.

Stoddard, C., & Thompson, D. (1996). Alcohol and the elderly: Special concerns for counseling professionals, *Alcoholism Treatment Quarterly, 14*(4), 59-69.

Substance Abuse and Mental Health Services Administration (SAMHSA) (2004). Substance abuse among older adults: Treatment Improvement Protocol (TIP) Series Number 26. United States Department of Health and Human Services, Rockville, MD.

U.S. Bureau of the Census (2000). Projected population of the United States, by age and sex: 2000-2050. Retrieved Jan. 2, 2004, from http://www.census.gov/ipc/www/usinterimproj/natprojtab02a.pdf

Vetere, A., & Henley, M. (2001). Integrating couples and family therapy into a community alcohol service: A pantheoretical approach. *Journal of Family Therapy, 23*, 85-101.

Westermeyer, J. (1991). Historical and social context of psychoactive substance disorders. In R. Francis & S. Miller (Eds.), *Clinical textbook of addictive disorders* (pp. 23-42). New York: Guilford.

Whitchurch, G., & Constantine, L. (1993). Systems theory. In P. Boss, W. Doherty, & R. LaRossa (Eds.), *Sourcebook of family theories and methods: A contextual approach.* (pp. 325-352). New York: Plenum.

Wilsnack, R., Vogeltanz, N., Wilsnack, S., & Harris, R. (2000). Gender differences in alcohol consumption and adverse drinking consequences: Cross-cultural patterns. *Addiction, 95*(2), 251-265.

doi:10.1300/J020v25n01_04

Family Motivation to Change: A Major Factor in Engaging Alcoholics in Treatment

James Garrett, CSW

Judith Landau, MB, ChB, DPM

SUMMARY. Family Motivation to Change can best be understood as the combined forces operating within a family guiding it towards maintaining survival in the face of serious threat, and towards healing when threat is removed. Exploring what happens to families during major disaster allowed the authors to step back into the grief that initiates the problem. The authors discovered that the force driving a family towards health is the same force that drove them to the initial adaptive behavior where a family member becomes addicted in an attempt to keep the family close, preventing them from feeling the pain of intense loss and sorrow. Once this has happened, the driving force of health and healing, "Family Motivation to Change," pushes, frees, or allows a member of the family, a natural change agent or Family Link to lead the family out of grief and addiction into health and recovery. doi:10.1300/J020v25n01_05 *[Article copies available for a fee from The Haworth Document Delivery Service: 1-800-HAWORTH. E-mail*

James Garrett is affiliated with Linking Human Systems, LLC, Albany, New York.
Judith Landau is affiliated with Linking Human Systems, LLC, Boulder, Colorado.
Address correspondence to: Judith Landau, Linking Human Systems, LLC, 503 Kalmia Avenue, Boulder, CO 80304 (E-mail: JLandau@LinkingHumanSystems.com).

[Haworth co-indexing entry note]: "Family Motivation to Change: A Major Factor in Engaging Alcoholics in Treatment." Garrett, James, and Judith Landau. Co-published simultaneously in *Alcoholism Treatment Quarterly* (The Haworth Press, Inc.) Vol. 25, No. 1/2, 2007, pp. 65-83; and: *Familial Responses to Alcohol Problems* (ed: Judith L. Fischer, Miriam Mulsow, and Alan W. Korinek) The Haworth Press, Inc., 2007, pp. 65-83. Single or multiple copies of this article are available for a fee from The Haworth Document Delivery Service [1-800-HAWORTH, 9:00 a.m. - 5:00 p.m. (EST). E-mail address: docdelivery@haworthpress.com].

Available online at http://atq.haworthpress.com
doi:10.1300/J020v25n01_05

KEYWORDS. Family motivation, motivation to change, breaking the intergenerational cycle, alcoholism in the family, addiction, concerned other, intervention, ARISE, invitational intervention, Transitional Family Therapy, treatment engagement, transitional pathway, transitional conflict, Family Link

INTRODUCTION

The family is the core unit of social relationships across all cultures. It is difficult to conceive of a culture surviving without the family. "The family is the natural context for both growth and healing–The family is the natural group which over time has evolved patterns of interacting. These patterns make up the family structure, which governs the functioning of family members, delineating their range of behavior and facilitating their interaction. A viable form of family structure is needed to perform the family's essential tasks of supporting individuation while providing a sense of belonging" (Minuchin & Fishman, 1981, page 112). For the purpose of this paper, family is defined as a domestic group of people, or a number of domestic groups, linked through descent (demonstrated or stipulated) from a common ancestor, marriage, or other committed coupling, legal or informal adoption, or through the choice to become kin to each other. It includes the extended intergenerational family network, by blood or choice, in its broadest sense. Stressors, such as untimely death, massive or unpredictable loss, cultural conflict, and unresolved grief, result in families getting off track from healthy functioning. In such situations, individual family members can become "symptomatic" and develop behaviors that are initially designed to protect the family from pain, keep families close, and help rebuild homeostatic functioning (Haley, 1980; Stanton, 1977). These adaptive behaviors later develop into destructive patterns that can be transmitted across generations, ultimately preventing the family from moving from one family life cycle stage to the next stage (Landau, 1982; Landau-Stanton, 1985; Landau, Garrett, et al., 2000). Alcoholism is known to be a risk associated with an increase in family stressors (Johnson, Richter, McLellan, & Kleber, 2002).

Studies of Jewish holocaust survivor families demonstrate how alcoholism results from disruption of family connectedness, family continuity and cultural transition. The rate of alcoholism in Jewish families prior to World War II was extremely low, while research after World War II shows alcoholism rates in subsequent generations of Jewish families that approach those in the population at large. This increase relates to the disruption in traditional family functioning, forced migration, conflicts in cultural transition and the significant number of holocaust related deaths. (McGoldrick, Pearce and Giordano, 1982; Perel & Saul, 1989). Addiction in refugee populations is approximately 30% higher than the general population (Landau & Saul, 2004; Landau, 2005). If increased family stressors and unresolved transitional conflict are related to the development of symptomatic behavior in individual family members, then a decrease in stressors and resolution of transitional conflict is likely to result in the return of competent family functioning and healthier individual functioning.

The concept, "Family Motivation to Change," presented in this paper, is based on the belief in the inherent competence and resilience of families. Alcoholism affects the family, and the family can positively affect recovery from alcoholism. Applying engagement and treatment methods for alcoholism based on this concept has been shown to improve treatment engagement, retention and outcome (Landau et al., 2004; Stanton & Shadish, 1998; Galanter, 1993). In addition to describing the concept, one of its practical applications for engaging resistant alcoholics in treatment will be presented in illustration.

THE FAMILY IN TRANSITION

Family Transitions

Transitional Family Therapy, the theoretical model on which our thinking is based, views the family as intrinsically competent, resilient and healthy and the family can be a resource for individuals in times of stress (Landau-Stanton, 1986; Watson & McDaniel, 1998; Walsh, 2003). Our goal is to empower families to identify resources that they can use to cope with life's challenges, including the important life cycle transitions or losses that confront them. Although change is a natural part of living, experiencing multiple transitions, typically 3 or more (even normal, predictable life-cycle events such as the birth of a baby, promotion of a breadwinner, or the death of an elder) within a short period of time can create stress (Boss, 2001; Figley & McCubbin, 1983; Garmezy & Rutter, 1983). It is during these times that families are likely to develop problems, exhibit symptoms, and need help. Accordingly, it is vital that therapists using Transitional Family Therapy approach individuals and families with the attitude that, given a set of tools and some brief therapeutic assistance, families are capable of designing effective solutions to their problems, rather than viewing them as "broken" and in need of lifelong hand-holding. This guiding principle forms the basis of "Family Motivation to Change."

We often refer to Transitional Family Therapy as a form of "brief intermittent therapy," since families work through a crisis, develop their own set of tools, learn to access their inherent resources, and develop a sense of competence, hope and faith in themselves. For the most part, this therapy enables them to deal with future challenges and life cycle transitions unassisted. However, there may be times when there have been a number of life cycle and other stressors in a short period of time, where a few family therapy sessions are once again helpful.

Transitional Conflict

In times of stress or upheaval, the response from molecular to interpersonal to societal level, is to disconnect or dissociate. During such times, the Transitional Pathway–the fragile but essential line connecting individuals' and families' past, present and future–can easily become disrupted and asynchrony between the rate and direction with which individual family members adjust to change results in "Transitional Conflict" (Landau-Stanton, 1990). The stress of transitional conflict, especially when upheaval is rapid or traumatic, such as when the natural direction of the life cycle is disrupted (e.g., untimely death like the death of an infant or child), or when resources are insufficient to balance the stresses (Hobfoll, 1989; Landau-Stanton & Clements, 1993) results in one of more members of the family becoming symptomatic. Transitional Family Therapy with adolescent alcohol abusers has been tested by Stanton using the *Transitional Family Therapy Treatment Manual for Use With Adolescent Alcohol Abuse and Dependence* (National Institute of Alcohol Abuse and Alcoholism, 1999; Landau & Garrett, 1998). The data from this study are currently in analysis.

Symptom as Adaptation: Intergenerational Transmission

Left unaddressed, transitional conflict arising from migration, rapid or unpredictable transitions, traumatic loss, and grief can lead to a variety of symptoms, including addiction, depression and suicidality, violence, post-traumatic stress, and risk-taking behaviors, including those that can lead to HIV/AIDS (Landau & Saul, 2004). For example, within one year after September 11th, 2001, there was a 31% increase in the rate of substance abuse and addiction in New York City and its immediate sur-roundings–approximating the addiction statistics of uprooted persons around the world (Johnson, Richter, McLellan & Kleber, 2002). At times of overwhelming grief, families find ways of compensating and staying close together, often without conscious intent. Frequently, one member of the family will begin to use alcohol or other substances, or exhibit other symptoms that serve the dual purpose of drawing the family's at-tention away from the grief and holding the family together to deal with the problems arising from the new problem behavior or symptoms. The result is that the family is unable to process their current transitions, re-maining locked in the transitional conflict of the moment. Since this maintains their closeness, it helps to assuage the grief and reduce the pain. When the symptoms or alcohol use are reduced, the pain and grief return, reinforcing the need for the problem. The addiction cycle is set, and is often transmitted across generations until the family grieving is resolved, the symptom has become redundant, and healing can occur (Landau, 1979, Landau, 1981; Landau & Stanton, 1990; Landau, Garrett, et al., 2000; Landau, 2004a; Landau, 2004b).

Family Resilience

When people are able to access past resilience by being in touch with their history, they can understand that the intergenerational history of alcoholism described above might well have been started as an attempt at adaptation to loss in order to protect the family from pain and to keep them together until their grief was resolved. This knowledge frees the current generation from guilt, shame, and the inevitability of a future locked into alcoholism. Hope is returned. They are able to reconnect their transitional pathways, knowing where they came from and where they are now. This allows them to recognize and utilize biological, psy-chological, social, and spiritual resources, making informed choices about what to keep from their past to draw on for the future and what to leave behind (Landau-Stanton & Clements, 1993). This is particularly relevant for practitioners dealing with alcoholism because the prevalent notion in the field is that patients struggling with recovery from alcoholism should be kept at a distance from their families. In exploring how families access and maintain resilience and competence across time, we examined the impact of attachment or connectedness to family and culture of origin in a series of women. The more connected they were, the less likely they were to take sexual risks. One of the measures was their knowledge of family stories, and even if those were problematic, it was still more protective than knowing no stories at all (Landau, Cole, Tuttle, Clements, & Stanton, 2000; Tuttle, Landau, Stanton, King, & Frodi, 2004). Other research indicates that strong social relationships and support can provide health protection, and that lacking these connections can compromise health (House, Landis, & Umberson, 1988; Rankin & Fukuoka, 2003).

Family Connectedness

The connection of the alcoholic to his/her family of origin is well documented (Stanton & Shadish, 1997). In fact, contrary to the common perception in the field, alcoholics care about their families and their families care about them. They remain very closely connected; in fact more closely connected than the general population. Averaging several studies, it appears that 9% of nonaddicts tend to call their families daily while addicted persons maintain daily contact with their families at a rate of approximately 57% in the US, 62% in England, 80% in Thailand and Italy, and 67% in Puerto Rico (Perzel & Lamon, 1979; Vaillant, 1995).

INDIVIDUAL MOTIVATION TO CHANGE

Prochaska and DiClemente's Stages of Change model represents six individual motivational stages that explain how an individual progresses from preparing for change to eventually taking action to change addictive behaviors and move into long-term recovery (Prochaska, DiClemente, & Norcross, 1992). This paper focuses on how Family Motivation to Change addresses the goal of getting a resistant alcoholic into treatment. *Family Motivation to Change* positively influences all six of the Stages of Change. We will, however, discuss only the first two stages of Prochaska and DiClimente's Individual Motivation to change, because these are the two on which Family Motivation to Change primarily impacts.

Stages of Change starts with Pre-contemplation, where the individual is too unwilling, unknowing or unable to acknowledge that the drinking problem requires a change in drinking behavior. Contemplation, the next stage, is where the individual recognizes that the drinking is a problem and may require a change in behavior, but is not ready to take action. These two stages are marked by denial of a problem, resistance to getting help and significant ambivalence. It is at these initial stages that we believe our Invitational Intervention method for engaging alcoholics in treatment, ARISE, A Relational Intervention Sequence for Engagement operates (Garrett, Landau-Stanton, Stanton, Stellato-Kabat, & Stellato-Kabat, 1997; Garrett et al., 1998; Garrett et al.,1999; Garrett & Landau, 1999; Landau, Garrett, et al., 2000).

FAMILY MOTIVATION TO CHANGE

Background and Philosophy

Family Motivation to Change can best be understood as the combined forces operating within a family that guide it towards maintaining survival in the face of serious threat, and health and sustained functioning when threat is removed. The authors have studied this process as it pertains to not only getting a loved one into alcoholism treatment, but also to enhance health-seeking, or reduce risk-taking, behaviors, in such areas as: sexual risk-taking for HIV-AIDS prevention; domestic violence; treatment and medication compliance for chronic and life threatening illness. We have termed this survival drive of the family "Family Motivation to Change" (Landau et al., 2004).

Exploring what happened to families during major disaster, allowed the authors to take a step back into the grief that initiated the problem (Landau & Garrett, 2005). We discovered that the force that drives a family towards health is the same force that drove them to the initial adaptive behavior described above where a family member becomes addicted in an attempt to keep the family close and to prevent them from feeling the pain of intense loss and sorrow. Eventually, the focus on the problems caused by the individual's alcoholism slows the process of successfully completing normal family life cycle transitions until the grief is resolved.

Once this has happened, the driving force of health and healing, "Family Motivation to Change," pushes, frees, or allows a member of the family, a natural change agent or Family Link to lead the family out of grief and addiction and into health and recovery (Landau, 1979, Landau, 1982; Landau-Stanton & Clements, 1993; Landau, 2004a).

Operational Process

The following section addresses how Family Motivation to Change is operationalized by families to get a loved one into alcoholism treatment. The process is typically activated by one member of the family who has the interest, motivation, strength, credibility and cross-generational knowledge of the family to act as a "Family Link" in starting and coordinating the process. Below are some of the key elements that operate on conscious and sub-conscious levels.

First Protecting and Then Healing the Family

The initial protection of the family starts unconsciously as one member of the family is drawn to offer him/herself as the sacrifice to serve as the diversion for a loved one from acute pain and grief, as discussed above. The motivating force functions to prevent the loved one from suffering grief to the extent that s/he might choose to join those lost in death. Each time that the alcoholic starts to succeed at a job, at leaving home, or at any other life cycle transition, the depression, grief, or overwhelming loss of the person s/he was protecting is likely to return. At this point, the alcoholic is highly likely to relapse, to save the loved one once again. It is only once the grief is resolved throughout the extended family that the alcoholic can succeed to traverse the life cycle transition with success and move into recovery for the long-term. At this stage, the same protective driving Family Motivation to Change force serves to bring first one, then the rest of the family into recovery. Continued, unresolved grief, results in the alcoholism being transmitted across and down the generations until the grief is resolved, and a family member leads the family into healing as described above.

Breaking the Intergenerational Cycle of Alcoholism

The intergenerational cycle of alcoholism can be broken by any member of the family. This happens in a number of different ways. It might be that an alcoholic decides that s/he is "sick and tired of being sick and tired," or a Concerned Other member of the family decides, "I'm not going to let this disease take any more members of my family," or a mother determines that she is not going to allow her sons to suffer as their father and grandfather did. The family members concerned are not aware of the underlying factors of resolved or unresolved grief, but are acting out of their commitment and Motivation to Change.

Completing the Transitional Task for "Peace of Mind"

As people approach vulnerable times in their lives, either through aging, illness, or trauma, and are reminded of their mortality, they start to focus on what they want to accomplish before they die. To quote an elderly patient, "I want peace of mind, heart and soul before leaving this earth and facing my maker. I want to see my sons in recovery and know that my grandchildren will not suffer as alcoholics like my husband and my sons." For many, it might mean completing a life cycle transition such as leaving home, giving a daughter permission to marry or have a child, or completing unresolved grief.

Getting a Loved One Back

Have you ever asked a family member who came to you for help related to an alcoholic to describe what the alcoholic loved one was like before the alcohol and/or drug use started? Have you ever had family members say to you, "It feels like I have lost my daughter," or "That is not my father anymore; he was never like that before the drinking got worse?" What each family member will describe is the memory of their loved one's functioning before alcoholism, and how the individual changed over time as the process of addiction became more and more intrusive, eventually changing thought patterns, attitudes and behaviors. Whether conscious or not, the family wants their alcoholic member "back the way s/he was." This longing is a powerful motivator for change and a powerful motivator for the family to be interested in "family recovery." Viewed this way, it is no longer an individual problem. It is a family problem and family recovery becomes the goal.

Preventing More Loss

Families are acutely aware of the risk of losing their loved one through risky behavior and this acts as a powerful element in Family Motivation to Change. The intense connectedness of family members that starts at the time of the first family member becoming alcoholic is an indicator of the life cycle stage at which the original stress precipitated the transitional conflict where the family became "stuck." This "stuckness" prevents further loss by holding family members close together until the grieving is done as described in an above section. Family connectedness is also the key dynamic that mobilizes family members to serve as effective "Family Links" allowing clinicians to "coach" them and their alcoholic loved ones to enter treatment and continue in recovery. This is in effect, "Family Motivation to Change" in action and is essential in the achievement of long-term commitment to growth and sustained change.

APPLICATION OF FAMILY MOTIVATION TO CHANGE TO THE PRE-CONTEMPLATION AND CONTEMPLATION STAGES OF CHANGE AND ON TO ACTION

Engaging alcoholics and drug addicts is a major challenge to the addictions treatment field: Less than 10% of addicted individuals ever get into treatment (Kessler et al., 1994). ARISE is a 3-Level method designed to use the motivation of family members to get a resistant individual with a drinking problem started in treatment. It is designed to maximize the efforts of the family (defined in the ARISE model as those members in the natural support system that are identified by the "First Caller") while minimizing the time and effort of the professional. The guiding principle is to stop at the first level that works. Level 1 uses motivational techniques designed specifically for telephone coaching, but they can also be applied to face-to-face sessions. We help the "First Caller" establish a basis of hope, identify whom to invite to the initial intervention meeting, design a strategy to mobilize the group, teach techniques to successfully invite the alcoholic to the first meeting, and get a commitment from all invited individuals to attend the initial meeting regardless of whether or not the alcoholic attends. Level 2 follows, if treatment does not start during Level 1. Typically, in Level 2, between two to five face-to-face sessions are held, with or without the alcoholic present, to mobilize the intervention network in developing motivational strategies to attain the goal of treatment engagement. Very few families (less than 2%) need to proceed to Level 3. In Level 3, family and friends set limits and consequences for the alcoholic in a loving and supportive way. By the time the intervention network gets to this point, the alcoholic has been given and has refused many opportunities to enter treatment. Because the alcoholic has been invited to each of the intervention network meetings, this final limit setting approach is a natural consequence, does not come as a surprise, and is often almost welcomed.

A recent trial of the ARISE Intervention showed that 83% of severely addicted alcoholics and substance abusers enrolled in treatment or attended self-help meetings following the intervention (Landau et al., 2004). Half of those who entered treatment did so within 1 week of the initial call from a concerned family member or friend, and 84% did so within 3 weeks. Preferred substance of abuse did not have any impact on engagement rate, nor on the level of the intervention at which engagement occurred. The engagement rate did not differ across demographic variables such as age, gender, or race. Finally, the study showed, professional therapists spent an average of less than an hour and a half coaching concerned friends and family members to mobilize their networks to motivate addicted subjects to enter treatment. Before it can be claimed with more certainty that the engagement numbers are reliable, replication by other investigators would be desirable.

The First Call

In the Pre-contemplation and Contemplation Stages of Change, the individual with a drinking problem is either unable or unwilling to see the problem and initiate a commitment to change. The ARISE method encourages clinicians to take a phone call from a concerned "First Caller" who is asking for help to get a resistant loved one into treatment. This initial request for help may also be done in a face-to-face interview. The ARISE method has a "First Call" protocol and specific coaching techniques that help focus and mobilize the "First Caller" into action (Garrett and Landau, 1999). The "First Caller" is coached as a "Family Link" to understand that: (a) s/he has done the right thing to reach out for help; (b) there is a method that has proven successful at getting resistant alcoholics into treatment; (c) it is important to mobilize as many family members and Concerned Others as possible to meet and focus on getting the alcoholic into treatment; (d) the process of an Invitational Intervention is done with love and respect, and (e) s/he no longer has to deal with the alcoholic one-on-one. There are times when it is appropriate for another person to join with the "First Caller" so the two individuals become "Co-Family Links." For instance, if a "First Caller" were a sibling of an alcoholic, it might be beneficial if the partner of the alcoholic became actively involved as a "Co-Family Link." An initial meeting is set up and the "First Caller" is coached on how to invite the alcoholic to that first meeting. There is no need for the alcoholic to sign a Release of Information form in order to have the initial meeting because this individual is not a client in treatment at the point of the "First Call" and at the time of the initial meeting. Contrary to what most clinicians believe, our research shows that 55% of the time the alcoholic shows up for the first meeting and by the end of 3-5 meetings, 83% of alcoholics have entered treatment (Landau et al., 2004).

These intervention meetings build on Family Motivation to Change and exert pressure on the unmotivated alcoholic (in the Pre-contemplation or Contemplation Stage of Change) to enter treatment. The power and strength of the family to provide motivation and support for the resistant alcoholic is unparalleled. No one else in the alcoholic's life has such a vested interest in, and long-term commitment to, his/her well-being. The statement of that love, concern, interest and support to make changes coming from a group of committed family and friends is a powerful motivator to help the unmotivated alcoholic move from Pre-contemplation to Contemplation and into treatment. Ongoing intervention network meetings, taking place after the alcoholic has entered treatment, result in a continuity of accountability with the alcoholic for continuing the difficult work required once treatment has begun. Research has demonstrated that there is a correlation between family involvement and longer term retention in treatment. The longer the time spent in treatment the better the outcome. (Conner et al., 1998; Stanton & Shadish, 1997).

Case Example

The authors are currently consulting in Kosova[1] to assist in the design and implementation of the Addiction Education, Resource and Tertiary Treatment Center in Pristina, Kosova, and the development of country-wide addiction services for Kosova–the first addiction treatment system in that country. The following case example demonstrates Family Motivation to Change in a cross-cultural context. Many of the cases coming into the Addictions Treatment Center are related to trauma and loss associated with the war and ethnic cleansing. Because there is little inter-generational history of alcoholism in the Kosovar families, since the predominant culture is secular Islam, the situation presents a unique opportunity to witness how families get off track and how alcoholism develops as an adaptation to major trauma and loss, before being transmitted into future generations. The following case example demonstrates this process.

Sanja is a 17-year-old female living with her widowed 46-year-old father, Jusuf. Sanja is the youngest of 3 children and was 11 years old when the war broke out in Kosova. Both parents were college educated. Her father worked as an engineer for an electrical plant and her mother was an elementary school teacher. The family valued education and placed a high expectation on completing college. The family lived in Prishtina, the capital of Kosova.

When the war broke out, the electrical power plant in which Sanja's father worked was destroyed. Sanja's mother was taken from their home and was later found dead. Jusuf went into a serious depression after the death of his wife and continues to experience problems with depression, including an inability to work. Up to the age of 15, Sanja was described as a talented student with a keen interest in mathematics and chemistry. Sanja began to exhibit acting out behaviors that included: skipping school, not coming home at night, sexual risk-taking, not doing home-work, defiance towards her father, mood changes and a change in her peer group to older youths known to be heavy drinkers and drug users. Jusuf could not handle his daughter's defiant behavior and the result was increased arguing and fighting between them.

Sanja was hospitalized overnight for symptoms that resembled a drug overdose, but she vehemently denied any drug use at the time of this incident. Sanja continued to exhibit out of control behaviors, con-sistently protesting that she did not drink alcohol or use drugs. Jusuf called the Addictions Treatment Center to find out what he could do to get help for his daughter. He was coached, using ARISE protocols, to approach his daughter, with love rather than threats or anger, about his growing concern for her well-being. He let her know that he would not tolerate her continued acting out and that he had set up an appointment at a treatment facility and would like her to accompany him, but that he would be going to the session regardless of whether or not she decided to attend. (Jusuf applied the driving force of Family Motivation to Change to get his resistant daughter Sanja started in treatment in an effort to get his beloved daughter back and to prevent further loss.)

In the first meeting, attended by Jusuf and his daughter Sanja, the genogram and timeline revealed that Jusuf and Sanja had suffered multi-ple losses. Not only had Jusuf lost his wife, and Sanja her mother, but Jusuf's mother (Sanja's grandmother–who had moved in with him to help with Sanja), had died as well the following year. Sanja had, there-fore, lost two key women in her life within one year. She had also witnessed her father going into a serious depression because of their deaths. Sanja was strongly denying any alcohol or drug use, in spite of a prior hospitalization for a suspected overdose. When Sanja was asked if she worried about her father she softened, starting to cry and told us the history of his depression and how much she constantly worried about him. It was clear that she understood the impact of loss on his functioning.

From a family life cycle point of view, it is clear that Sanja was caught in a dilemma regarding her successfully leaving home. Even though her leaving would be natural and age appropriate, there was a level at which she realized that her father would experience yet another loss because she was all he had left. Her leaving home would likely result in increasing her father's depression. How could she bring harm to someone she loved so much? Not being able to verbalize those thoughts and feelings, even to herself, Sanja started acting out by using alcohol and drugs. This created tension between her and her father, and he kicked her out of their home. Sanja's dilemma about leaving her father and causing more loss in his life was resolved.

Once the clinician shared her perception of the situation, Sanja admitted to her alcohol and drug use, and even though she did not fully understand the impact of her actions, she was able to state, "I was hoping that he would end up hating me and would be happy to see me out of the house." After Sanja agreed to stop her drug and alcohol use (moving from Pre-contemplation into Action), we proceeded to: (a) help Jusuf see how much Sanja loved him; (b) encourage Sanja to see that she did not have to sacrifice herself in order to leave home successfully; (c) ensure that Jusuf received treatment for depression; (d) work with father and daughter to address the "normal" loss of a child leaving home, and, at the same time, (e) plan for supporting a continued family life-cycle appropriate relationship between the two.

This adaptive behavior by Sanja was designed to protect her father from experiencing another loss and increased depression, and also to take his mind off the multiple losses in the family and his unresolved grief. If unaddressed, one might project how this "adaptive" behavior could have resulted in her "pseudo-individuation," and the development of alcoholism with the unresolved losses carrying over into the next and future generations. If Jusuf were to die before these issues were resolved and while she was still out of the house and using alcohol and drugs, Sanja would likely feel guilty that her father had died alone and grieving. Her guilt would be increased because of her not being there for him when he really needed her, and for having made him suffer yet another loss. This lack of resolution of the increasing losses might also result in her increased alcohol and drug use at this time.

CONCLUSION:
PRACTICAL APPLICATION AND FUTURE IMPLICATIONS FOR TREATMENT AND TREATMENT OUTCOME

In conclusion, Family Motivation to Change is essentially the driving force in families that activates resilience and moves them towards health. During times of adversity, loss and trauma, members of a family may become symptomatic, but the family as a whole retains the capacity to heal. We believe that both families and professionals can tap into this resource by trusting in the inherent competence and resilience of families to overcome the despair, shame and guilt of the alcoholic process and access Family Motivation to Change. This driving force can be harnessed to mobilize their support system to motivate alcoholic loved ones into treatment. In fact, we believe that Family Motivation to Change is the primary factor that frees the alcoholic to move from Pre-contemplation into Contemplation and then into Action.

ARISE (A Relational Intervention Sequence for Engagement) is one of the practical methods that applies Family Motivation to Change to guide and coach families into successfully getting a resistant alcoholic loved one into treatment. Its unusual rate of success can only be attributed to the initiative, dedication, caring, concern and insight of the family members and concerned others in the support systems involved in this Invitational Intervention method.

There is considerable evidence that involvement of families in alcohol treatment has a positive impact on treatment retention (Steinglass, 1987; O'Farrell, 1992; O'Farrell & Fals-Stewart, 1999; Carroll, 1997; Loneck, Garrett, & Banks, 1997). In addition, several studies point to improved treatment outcomes with higher treatment retention rates (Stark, Campbell & Brinkerhoff, 1990; Stark, 1992). It might therefore seem reasonable to hypothesize that applying Family Motivation to Change in order to maximize family involvement from the very beginning of the treatment engagement process might well improve treatment outcome and long-term recovery.

NOTE

1. Kosova Ministry of Health and European Agency for Reconstruction (EAR): Establishment of an Addiction Education, Resource and Tertiary Treatment Center in Pristina, Kosova, and Country-Wide Addiction Services for Kosova. PI: J. Landau; Co-PI: J. Garrett.

REFERENCES

Boss, P. (2001). *Family stress management: a contextual approach.* Thousand Oaks, CA: Sage.

Carroll, K. M. (1997). Enhancing retention in clinical trials of psychosocial treatment: Practical strategies. In L. S. Onken, J. D. Blaine, & J. J. Boren (Eds.), *Beyond the therapeutic alliance: keeping the drug-dependent individual in treatment. NIDA Research Monograph 165* (pp. 11). Rockville, MD: U.S. Department of Health and Human Services, National Institutes of Health.

Conner, K. R., Shea, R. R., McDermott, M. P., Grolling, R., Tocco, R. V., & Baciewicz, G. (1998). The role of multifamily therapy in promoting retention to treatment of alcohol and cocaine dependence. *American Journal of Addictions, 71*(1), 61-73.

Figley, C. R., & McCubbin, H. I. (Eds.) (1983). *Stress and the family: Vol. 2. Coping with normative transitions.* New York: Brunner/Mazel.

Galanter, M. (1993). *Network therapy for alcohol and drug abuse.* New York: Basic Books.

Garmezy, N., & Rutter, M. (1983). *Stress, coping & development in children.* NY: McGraw-Hill.

Garrett, J., Landau-Stanton, J., Stanton, M. D., Stellato-Kabat, J., & Stellato-Kabat, D. (1997). ARISE: A method for engaging reluctant alcohol- and drug-dependent individuals in treatment. *Journal of Substance Abuse Treatment, 13*(5), 1-14.

Garrett, J., Landau, J., Stanton, M. D., Baciewicz, G., Brinkman-Sull, D., & Shea, R. (1998). The ARISE intervention: Using family links to overcome resistance to addiction treatment. *Journal of Substance Abuse Treatment, 15*(2), 333-343.

Garrett, J., Stanton, M. D., Landau, J., Baciewicz, G., Brinkman-Sull, D., & Shea, R. (1999). The "Concerned Other" call: Using family links to overcome resistance to addiction treatment. *Substance Use and Misuse, 34*(3), 363-382.

Garrett, J., & Landau, J. (1999). *ARISE: A relational intervention sequence for engagement—training manual for certified ARISE interventionists.* Boulder, CO: Linking Human Systems.

Haley, J. (1980). *Leaving home.* New York: McGraw-Hill.

Hobfoll, S. E. (1989). Conservation of resources: A new attempt at conceptualizing stress. *American Psychologist, 44*, 513-524.

House, J. S., Landis, K. R., & Umberson, D. (1988). Social relationships and health. *Science, 241*, 540-545.

Johnson, P. B., Richter, L., McLellan, A. T., & Kleber, H. D. (2002). Alcohol use patterns before and after September 11. *American Clinical Laboratory, 21*(7), 25-27.

Kessler, R. C., McGonagle, K. A., Zhao, S., Nelson, C. B., Hughes, M., Eshleman, S., Wittchen, H. U., & Kendler, K. S. (1994). Lifetime and 12 month prevalence of DSM-III-R psychiatric disorders in the United States: Results from the National Comorbidity Survey. *Archives of General Psychiatry, 51*, 8-19.

Landau, J. (1979, July). *The black African family in transitional conflict.* Paper presented at the World Congress of the International Family Therapy Association, Tel Aviv, Israel.

Landau, J. (1981). Link therapy as a family therapy technique for transitional extended families. *Psychotherapeia*, October, 7(4), 382-390.

Landau, J. (1982). Therapy with families in cultural transition. In M. McGoldrick, J. K. Pearce, & J. Giordano (Eds.), *Ethnicity and family therapy*. New York: Guilford Press.

Landau, J. (2004a, March). *Family motivation to change using invitational intervention in substance abuse treatment*. Paper presented at the 14th World Congress of the International Family Therapy Association on Families in Times of Global Crisis, Istanbul, Turkey.

Landau, J. (2004b, September). *Family motivation to change: Families and therapists as partners for addiction recovery*. Paper presented at the Annual Conference of The American Association for Marriage and Family Therapy, Atlanta, GA.

Landau, J. (2005). El modelo LINC: una estrategia colaborativa para la resiliencia comunitaria. *Sistemas Familiares, 20*(3).

Landau, J., Cole, R., Tuttle, J., Clements, C. D., & Stanton, M. D. (2000). Family connectedness and women's sexual risk behaviors: Implications for the prevention/intervention of STD/HIV infection. *Family Process, 39*(4), 461-475.

Landau, J., & Garrett, J. (1998). *Transitional family therapy treatment manual for use with adolescent alcohol abuse and dependence*. Boulder, CO: Linking Human Systems, LLC.

Landau, J., & Garrett, J. (2005, June). *Family motivation to change and invitational intervention: The Kosovar experience*. Paper presented at the American Family Therapy Academy & 15th World Congress of the International Family Therapy Association, Washington, DC.

Landau, J., Garrett, J., Shea, R., Stanton, M. D., Baciewicz, G., & Brinkman-Sull, D. (2000). Strength in numbers: Using family links to overcome resistance to addiction treatment. *American Journal of Drug and Alcohol Abuse, 26*(3), 379-398.

Landau, J., & Saul, J. (2004). Facilitating family & community resilience in response to major disaster. In F. Walsh & M. McGoldrick (Eds.), *Living beyond loss 2nd Ed.* New York: Norton.

Landau, J., & Stanton, M. D. (1990). *Alcoholism and addiction within the family: intergenerational genesis, transmission, maintenance of symptoms, therapeutic implications*. Unpublished manuscript.

Landau, J., Stanton, M. D., Brinkman-Sull, D., Ikle, D., McCormick, D., Garrett, J., Baciewicz, G., Shea, R., & Wamboldt, F. (2004). Outcomes with *ARISE* approach to engaging reluctant drug-and alcohol-dependent individuals in treatment. *American Journal of Drug & Alcohol Abuse, 30*(4), 711-748.

Landau-Stanton, J. (1985). Adolescents, families, and cultural transition: A treatment model. In M. P. Mirkin & S. L. Koman (Eds.), *Handbook of adolescents and family therapy*. New York: Gardner Press, p. 363.

Landau-Stanton, J. (1986). Competence, impermanence, and transitional mapping: A model for systems consultation. In L.C. Wynne, S. McDaniel, & T. Weber (Eds.), *Systems consultations: A new perspective for family therapy* (pp. 253-269). New York: Guilford Press.

Landau-Stanton, J. (1990). Issues and methods of treatment for families in cultural transition. In M. P. Mirkin (Ed.), *Social & political contexts of family therapy* (pp. 251-275). Boston: Allyn & Bacon.

Landau-Stanton, J., & Clements, C. (1993). *AIDS, health and mental health: A primary sourcebook*. New York: Brunner/Mazel.

Loneck, B., Garrett, J., & Banks, S. (1997). Engaging and retaining women in outpatient alcohol and other drug treatment: The effect of referral intensity. *Health and Social Work, 22*(1), 38-46.

McGoldrick, M., Pierce, J. K., & Giordano, J. (Eds.). (1982). *Ethnicity and family therapy*. New York: Guilford Press.

Minuchin, S., & Fishman, H. (1981). *Family therapy techniques*. Cambridge, MA: Harvard University Press.

National Institute of Alcohol Abuse and Alcoholism (1999). Family and group therapies for adolescent alcohol abuse. (1 RO1 AA 12178-01). P. I., M. D. Stanton.

O'Farrell, T. J. (1992). Families and alcohol problems: An overview of treatment research. *Journal of Family Psychology, 5*, 339-359.

O'Farrell, T. J., & Fals-Stewart, W. (1999). Treatment models and methods: family models. In: McCrady, B. S., and Epstein, E. E., (Eds.), *Addictions: A comprehensive guidebook*. New York: Oxford Press.

Perel, E., & Saul, J. (1989). A family therapy approach to Holocaust survivor families. In P. Marcus, & A. Rosenberg (Eds.), *Healing their wounds: Psychotherapy with Holocaust survivors and their families*. New York: Praeger.

Perzel, J. F., & Lamon, S. (1979). *Enmeshment within families of polydrug abusers.* Paper presented at the National Drug Abuse Conference, New Orleans, August, 1979.

Prochaska, J. O., Di Clemente, C. C., & Norcross, J. C. (1992). In search of how people change: Applications to addictive behavior. *American Psychologist, 47*, 1102-1114.

Rankin, S. H., & Fukuoka, Y. (2003). Predictors of quality of life in women 1 year after myocardial infarction. *Progress in Cardiovascular Nursing, 18*(1): 6-12.

Seaburn, D., Landau-Stanton, J., & Horwitz, S. (1995). Core intervention techniques in family therapy process. In R. H. Mikesell, D. D. Lusterman, & S. H. McDaniel (Eds.), *Integrating family therapy: Handbook of family psychology and systems theory*. Washington, DC: American Psychological Association.

Stanton, M.D. (1977). The addict as savior: Heroin, death and the family. *Family Process, 16*(2), 191-197.

Stanton, M. D., & Shadish, W. R. (1997). Outcome, attrition and family/couples treatment for drug abuse: A meta-analysis and review of the controlled, comparative studies. *Psychological Bulletin, 122*(2), 170-191.

Stark, M. J. (1992). Dropping out of substance abuse treatment: A clinically oriented review. *Clinical Psychology Review, 12*, 93-116.

Stark, M. J., Campbell, B. K., & Brinkerhoff, C. V. (1990). "Hello, may we help you?" a study of attrition prevention at the time of the first phone contact with substance-abusing clients. *American Journal of Drug and Alcohol Abuse, 16*(1 & 2), 67-76.

Steinglass, P., Bennett, L, Wolin, S., & Reiss, D. (1987). *The alcoholic family*. New York: Basic Books.

Tuttle, J., Landau, J., Stanton, M. D., King, K., & Frodi, A. (2004). Intergenerational family relations and sexual risk behavior in young women. *The American Journal of Maternal Child Nursing, 29*(1), 56-61.

Vaillant, G. E. (1995). *The natural history of alcoholism revisited.* Cambridge, MA: Harvard University Press.

Walsh, F. (2003). Family resilience: A framework for clinical practice. *Family Process, 42*(1), 1-18.

Watson, W., & McDaniel, S. (1998) Assessment in transitional family therapy: The importance of context. In J. W. Barron (Ed.), *Making diagnosis meaningful: Enhancing evaluation and treatment of psychological disorders* (pp. 161-195). Washington, DC: American Psychological Association.

doi:10.1300/J020v25n01_05

Family Response to Adults and Alcohol

Robert Navarra, PsyD

SUMMARY. Studies indicate that couple and family relationships play a significant role in alcohol dependence and recovery processes, yet a relational framework in alcoholism treatment and research paradigms remains largely absent. Reciprocal, interactive dynamics between the alcoholic and couple-family relationships suggests the need for a more comprehensive conceptualization of alcoholism, inclusive of a relational perspective in addition to the current individual emphasis on abstinence as the defining measurement of successful treatment. Family variables, especially the couple relationship, underscore the importance of the concept of "couple recovery." Bridging the gap between individual and couple recovery requires: multiple levels of intervention, developmentally appropriate strategies through the stages of recovery, and openness to integrating various therapeutic approaches. The Couples Reciprocal Development Approach (CRDA), a theory of long-term couple recovery from alcoholism, identifies three distinct but interactive components of couple functioning. doi:10.1300/J020v25n01_06 *[Article copies available for a fee from The Haworth Document Delivery Service: 1-800-HAWORTH. E-mail address: <docdelivery@haworthpress.com> Website: <http://www.HaworthPress. com> © 2007 by The Haworth Press, Inc. All rights reserved.]*

KEYWORDS. Recovering couples, relational therapy and alcoholism, couples reciprocal development

---

Robert Navarra is Co-Founder and Acting Director of the Center for Couples in Recovery, Mental Research Institute (MRI), Palo Alto, California (E-mail: rnavarra@aol.com).

[Haworth co-indexing entry note]: "Family Response to Adults and Alcohol." Navarra, Robert. Co-published simultaneously in *Alcoholism Treatment Quarterly* (The Haworth Press, Inc.) Vol. 25, No. 1/2, 2007, pp. 85-104; and: *Familial Responses to Alcohol Problems* (ed: Judith L. Fischer, Miriam Mulsow, and Alan W. Korinek) The Haworth Press, Inc., 2007, pp. 85-104. Single or multiple copies of this article are available for a fee from The Haworth Document Delivery Service [1-800-HAWORTH, 9:00 a.m. - 5:00 p.m. (EST). E-mail address: docdelivery@haworthpress.com].

Available online at http://atq.haworthpress.com
© 2007 by The Haworth Press, Inc. All rights reserved.
doi:10.1300/J020v25n01_06

INTRODUCTION

The consequences of alcoholism äre pervasive and severe within the family (McCrady & Epstein, 1995; Moos & Moos, 1984; Rotunda, Scherer, & Imm, 1995; Steinglass, Bennett, Wolin, & Reiss, 1987) but disruptions in relational and family functioning as a result of alcoholism do not end with recovery; the aftereffects of years of alcoholism may still be evident in the couple-family system long after beginning recovery (Brown & Lewis, 1995, 1999; Usher, Jay, and Glass, 1982). Furthermore, studies suggest interactional processes between alcoholics and their family relationships–especially with family of origin and spouses–remain significant throughout addiction and recovery phases (Edwards & Steinglass, 1995; Humphreys, Moos, & Cohen, 1997; Navarra, 2002; Steinglass, Tislenko, & Reiss, 1985). Research on families and alcoholism validates Heath and Stanton's (1998) assertion that "Many other factors can also be critical (e.g., environmental, economic, cultural), but family variables hold a position of salience in the arena of addictive symptomology" (p. 496).

DIRECTIONS IN FAMILY STUDIES

Current family alcoholism research, evolving from the advances in behavioral and systemic theories of the 1980's and 1990's, characteristically focuses on three main areas of concern: the effect of alcoholism on the family, the role of the family in the etiology and progression of alcoholism, and the development of family-oriented treatment models to reduce drinking. While these studies add to the knowledge base of family therapy treatment for alcoholism, limitations are evident and underscore the need for new perspectives in families and addictions research.

First, comprehensive theories of addiction treatment and recovery require a long-term perspective (Collins, 1990; Jacob, 1992; McCrady & Epstein, 1995). McCrady (1990) concluded 15 years ago that treatment outcomes of behavioral interventions with couples beyond two years proved poor and statistically insignificant. Unfortunately, this statement is as true today as it was then. Likewise, well-constructed longitudinal studies on the effectiveness of systemic approaches are lacking.

Second, there are few qualitative studies on families and addictions. Qualitative analysis allows for conceptual density and complexity, a dynamic noticeably missing from current quantitative studies. Gilgun, Daly, and Handle (1992) argue for qualitative methods in the development of theory in family research, emphasizing grounded theory approaches in particular and view theory development as central to the very purpose of family research.

Third, measures for successful treatment outcomes limited to successful abstinence without reference to family functioning overlooks family variables, even though relational concerns remain central to alcoholic symptomology and recovery. Regrettably, the couple relationship and adjustment issues to addiction and recovery dynamics are rarely considered or evaluated in outcome measures. Currently, successful treatment outcomes are primarily determined by measures of reduced drinking or days of abstinence, an outcome measure problematic at two levels: (a) difficulties in the family continue or get worse after the alcoholic stops drinking (Brown & Lewis, 1995, 1999; Usher et al., 1982), and (b) even though the alcoholic stops drinking, the couple system remains essentially the same functionally and systemically. The "dry drunk" syndrome, or "white knuckle sobriety" refers to abstinence without recovery.

Research aimed at identifying and incorporating developmentally appropriate family-based interventions adjunctively with individual treatment follows as a logical next step in research. For example, current research indicates that working on intimacy and closeness for the couple in early recovery is contraindicated and could serve to undo individual recovery processes (Brown & Lewis, 1995, 1999). A more appropriate relational focus might include the following therapeutic approaches: providing a holding environment composed of supportive therapy, parent education, psychoeducation around addiction and recovery processes, and reinforcing individual work and 12-step participation. On the other hand, couples in long-term recovery may very well need help in developing intimacy and closeness. Finally, theories of couple recovery processes remain conspicuously absent in the addiction literature, especially research aimed toward bridging and integrating individual and couple recoveries.

RELATIONAL PERSPECTIVES IN ALCOHOLISM RESEARCH

Evolution in the field of alcoholism research and treatment over the last 60 years, with ever-increasing understanding and appreciation of the importance of family dynamics, presents a compelling argument for conceptualizing alcoholism assessment and treatment within a context of a relational perspective (Jacob, 1992; McCrady & Epstein, 1995; O'Farrell, 1992; Rotunda, Scherer, & Imm, 1995; Steinglass, 1976).

Humphreys, Moos, and Cohen (1997) found four factors associated with successful alcoholic remission measured at three- and eight-years after treatment. A summary of the results is as follows: (a) at the eight-year follow-up family relationship quality appears to be most predictive of remission, (b) short-term interventions have little long-term impact, (c) outpatient sessions sought in the first three years of recovery increased the likelihood of remission at the eight-year mark, (d) individuals who attended more Alcoholic Anonymous (AA) meetings in the first three years were more likely to remain in remission at eight-years and have lower levels of depression. The importance of satisfactory family relationships is underscored as the most predictive variable of long-term sobriety. Support from the family and from external sources (AA and outpatient psychotherapy) appear pivotal to successful long-term recovery.

A meta-analysis of 21 studies of treatment outcomes with family-involved alcoholism treatment approaches (Edwards and Steinglass, 1995) found family therapy effective in motivating the alcoholic into treatment, an outcome supported previously by O'Farrell (1992). However, family-involved treatment appears minimally more effective over time than individually-oriented treatment, with positive effects dissipating by year one post treatment, a result substantiated by Winters, Fals-Stewart, O'Farrell, Birchler, and Kelley (2000). In contrast to the disappointing treatment effectiveness of family therapy over time in the alcohol studies, Stanton and Shadish (1997) in a meta-analysis of studies across 1,571 cases of family-couples therapy with adult and adolescent drug abusers, found family therapy as more effective than individual and group counseling, with results still apparent even 4 years after treatment ended.

Combining and integrating individual and family treatment methodologies appears to maximize chances for long-term successful recovery. O'Farrell (1992) advocates development of a family therapy specialty, suggesting the title "Families and Addictions" with emphasis on "...the study of the role of the family in the etiology, course, treatment, and prevention of addictive behavior problems, to include problems with alcohol, drugs, smoking, and obesity" (p. 339).

INTERACTIONAL PERSPECTIVE

Family researchers have sought to understand the effect of the family (nuclear and extended) on the etiology and progression of alcoholism in one or more family members, and the impact of alcoholism on individual family members. The principle of the reciprocal relationship between the alcoholic and the family, usually extending beyond the nuclear family to include a multigenerational perspective of alcoholism, represents a framework for understanding both the progression of active alcoholism symptomology and for alcoholism recovery.

The couple sub-system holds a place of centrality within the family system. A theory of addiction and recovery processes without understanding the critical nature of the interplay, the reciprocity, between the individual alcoholic and the couple relationship misses the mark. A relational emphasis shifts the alcoholism research/treatment paradigm toward integration, consolidating intrapsychic with interpersonal dynamics into an overall theory of addiction and recovery processes.

Alcoholism sets in motion and delineates family regulatory mechanisms. A systemic perspective uncovers family defense mechanisms of denial and other enabling operations that help maintain alcoholic drinking. Families adapt and may attempt to explain away the alcoholic drinking or try to help the alcoholic moderate or control drinking, but these efforts are seldom successful, especially given the progressive nature of the alcoholism.

Conversely, the cost to the family of an alcoholic is high, affecting psychological health, relationships, and an increased risk for severe family dysfunction. Individual family members, whether or not they eventually develop their own alcoholism, have inherited an alcoholic legacy and an internalized sense of identity with alcohol that defines self and defines relationships with others. Disruptions in adult development, family functioning, and family life cycle due to alcoholism are central concerns in assessment and treatment. Alcoholic family systems are organized and function around alcohol (Brown & Lewis 1995; Steinglass et al., 1987; Usher et al., 1982), potentially affecting individual development in innumerable ways when considering the trauma of alcoholism and resultant marital and familial disruptions, attachment insecurities, and defensive mechanisms to cope and adapt to trauma.

The complexity and all-encompassing nature of addiction and recovery processes require a broad theoretical understanding. Multiple levels of intervention may include (a) biological, (b) psychological, (c) systemic, (d) interpersonal, and (e) social perspectives. A long-term outlook helps not only in viewing alcoholism across the life span, but also in conceptualizing and formulating treatment goals based on systemic and developmental issues. A relational component of addiction treatment includes consideration of such variables as: family organization around alcoholism; the impact of family history, especially alcoholism history; individual and interpersonal developmental processes, and an understanding of normal developmental recovery processes.

Application and integration of the reciprocal relationship between the alcoholic and co-alcoholic has not been applied to a systematic theory of treatment and recovery. Little attention has been paid to the concept of couple recovery despite what is now known about the effectiveness–and potential effectiveness–of couple-family treatment for alcoholism.

A systemic perspective analyzes interactions between parts and the "organized complexity" of the system as nonlinear in nature (Bertalanffy, 1969). The alcoholic couple as a dynamic, interactive system contains numerous variables and categories of organization around addiction and/or recovery processes. Assessing the interactive and nonlinear nature of individual and relationship recoveries anticipates possible problem areas. For example, studies indicate that the spouse plays a role in relapse and recovery (Fichter, Gylnn, Weyerer, & Liberman, 1997; O'Farrell, Hooley, Fals-Stewart, & Cutter, 1998). The circularity of the interactional perspective addresses both the substance issues and the state of the relationship between the alcoholic and partner, with awareness that one can not be considered without the other. Couple therapy can not and should not replace individual recovery; emphasis here is on the integration of couple with individual recoveries. Three recoveries are addressed simultaneously, each spouse's individual recoveries and the couple recovery. Limiting the focus to one component of the system, i.e., abstinence behaviors, without understanding its relationship to other components–such as spousal support, or the impact of an alcoholic legacy from the family of origin–becomes reductionistic, missing the bigger picture in the relationship between individual and couple processes.

THE COUPLE RECIPROCAL DEVELOPMENT APPROACH

Background

The Family Recovery Project (FRP) at the Mental Research Institute, directed by Stephanie Brown, Ph.D. and Virginia Lewis, Ph.D., began in 1989 with the goal of determining normal developmental processes in family and couple systems in recovery from alcoholism (Brown & Lewis, 1995, 1999). The Couples Focus Group, one component of the FRP, formed when three couples each with at least five years of recovery from alcoholism were invited by one of the researchers to participate in a one time meeting to discuss the impact of recovery on their relationships. At the end of the session the participants responded so enthusiastically to this unique opportunity to tell their story as a couple that they spontaneously and unanimously requested additional meetings. The group negotiated with Brown and Lewis to meet for two hours once a month for three months. Every three months, remarkably for over five years, the group renegotiated this agreement.

The researchers maintained a nondirective role in the structure and direction of the group, which remained a focus group, not a therapy group. The participants spoke about their evolving marital and family relationships in the context of their alcoholism and recovery histories. Additionally, ongoing and new issues were addressed as they unfolded, so that participants were not simply reporting their recovery histories, they shared current problems and triumphs in their individual lives, their marital lives, and in their family lives (both nuclear and extended families).

Each session was audiotaped and later analyzed utilizing grounded theory (Navarra, 2002). As opposed to descriptive studies which seek only to tell a story, or verificational methodologies with attachments to preconceived and predetermined biases, grounded theory methods are aimed at theory development based on a systematic approach to data collection and analysis. Theory evolves from the emerging data through the "constant comparison method," a coding technique in determining thematic consistency and relevance to the phenomena under study (Glaser & Strauss, 1967). The Couples Focus Group remained a naturalistic environment, affording the advantage of witnessing couples face passages of the family life cycle over time as events and transitions unfolded. Morgan (1997) advocates for less structured groups, especially when little is known about the area under study:

> What makes less structured focus groups such a strong tool for exploratory research is the fact that a group of interested participants can spark a lively discussion among themselves without much guidance from either the researcher's questions or the moderator's direction. In other words, if the goal is to learn something new from the participants, then it's best to let them speak for themselves. (p. 40)

The Center for Couples in Recovery (CCR), located at Mental Research Institute, was formed with the goal of continuing this ongoing research effort toward the development of an evolving theory of couple recovery. Couple recovery groups and individual couple therapy sessions are recorded and analyzed, adding to the growing body of data suggesting a predictable trajectory of long-term couple recovery processes.

A Theory of Long-Term Couple Recovery

The Couples Reciprocal Development Approach (CRDA), based on results from Couples Focus Group study, suggests a theoretical framework in conceptualizing long-term couple recovery processes. As an ongoing research project, CDRA is a work in progress, modifiable and evolving based on additional data.

Successful couple recovery from addiction involves more than couple adaptation to sobriety. Healthy couple development in ongoing recovery is distinguished from early recovery by emergent shifts in processes related to the capacity for deepened interpersonal relationships. Emphasis on individual growth and development now recede into the background as relationship patterns with children, parents, and spouse place more centrally in couple and family life. Fundamental intrapsychic and interpersonal issues dominate the developmental schemata of couple recovery as the couple members seek healthier relationships, and at the same time develop a stronger, more individuated sense of self. These evolving and unfolding issues include: (a) new identity formations; (b) restructuring of role relationships; (c) reordering of boundaries; (d) increased levels of working through attachment issues, especially with family of origin; (e) greater coping ability and tolerance for expression of emotional pain, most noticeably grief; and (f) a greater capacity to manage both individual and couple recoveries concurrently.

Three main components comprise the core areas of couple development: (a) centrality of the couple relationship identity, (b) integrating insights from the effect of family of origin issues on the relationship, and (c) the ability to foster an interdependent relationship. These areas of couple development are referred to respectively as "Shifting," "Intergenerational Reworking," and "Attending." Each component has multiple properties and operates in a nonlinear, interactional dynamic with the other components forming a nonlinear perspective on couple developmental. These distinct but overlapping phases of development collectively provide the framework for addressing multiple and simultaneous levels of individual and interpersonal processes. The degree of resolution and integration of these components is associated with the degree of successful couple recovery processes. A brief overview of the categories follows; quotations illustrate core concepts.

Shifting. Central reorganization of couple functioning begins with an orientation moving away from the exclusivity of individual recovery to an emphasis on couple identity formation. The couple relationship system, abandoned in early recovery in service to individual recovery now emerges into a place of primacy. In Shifting dramatic changes occur in definitions of the couple relationship, roles, and boundaries.

Mary describes her new recognition of an emerging identity as a recovering couple:

> Mary: I had an awareness just this past week when it was just Leo and me on vacation, that there are three recoveries going on: mine as alcoholic, Leo's as a person who had a relationship with an alcoholic, and then our relationship, which is a total entity.

In another session Mary speaks to the concept of couple development over time. Previously, Mary emphasized changes she experienced in her own development as a recovering alcoholic. In the group Mary stressed an increasing attentiveness to changes as a couple within the framework of a recovering couple identity.

> Mary: ...and we got to experience every day, every minute, two different people, two people [emphasized] in recovery. It becomes different the further we get from the drinking. There is not nearly as much drama in our lives. Even three or four years ago, it's interesting to me how things change.... I do feel like I can look back at phases in our history as a couple in recovery and see very different experiences in the way we interact with one another, and the way we make decisions, and the way we handle situations, even thinking back to two years ago, how I felt about my family.

In active alcoholic family systems boundaries are blurred and/or rigidly exclusionary (Preli, Protinsky, & Cross, 1990; Rotunda, Scherer, & Imm, 1995). With the progression of addictive symptomology couples adapt to the alcoholic's increasing loss of control with the alcoholic's spouse either withdrawing and or attempting to compensate for the lack of the alcoholic's participation in family and couple life.

Entrance into recovery demarcates enormous developmental shifts in the marital system. The enmeshed active alcoholic marital system, typified by the alcoholic's preoccupation with alcohol and the partner's preoccupation with the alcoholic's drinking, give way to increased differentiation in recovery. A culture of recovery replaces isolation and breaks through the closed system of active alcoholism. Emphasis on individual work and differentiation is essential in early recovery; 12-step programs like AA and Al-Anon help facilitate this process by providing tools for self-awareness, self-care, and taking responsibility for self.

While in early recovery the relational developmental transition could be described as "A couple in search of individual identities," in ongoing recovery the developmental shift moves to "Individuals in search of a couple identity." This transition relates directly to the central importance of the concept of couple recovery. All the alcoholic members in the Couples Focus Group regularly attended Alcoholic Anonymous (AA) while the nonalcoholic spouses had varying degrees of involvement in Al-Anon. Few research couples at CCR to date have attended Recovering Couples Anonymous (RCA), a 12-step program based on the principles of AA and focused on helping couples identify and change unhealthy relationship patterns. Group members validated the importance of their individual 12-step programs but admitted these programs did not address their marital relationship, an issue increasingly problematic in long-term recovery.

> Nan: I have trouble with a 12-step program as working on your marriage per se because that's where we got into it, that's when we got into dueling programs. We truly felt we needed an outside facilitator.
>
> Leo: I think what I miss in some 12-step meetings is this kind of stuff [referring to content covered in focus group] what is talked about, because these kinds of problems that come up are the problems that I also experience...these kind of topics do not come up in those meetings...
>
> Kyle: So it has been a way of sort of moving outside, of moving sort of beyond AA into something closer to my own sort of domestic life, my own family life, because we don't go to meetings together.
>
> Mary: AA is wonderful. But remember AA is mine, and Al-Anon is his. What do we have for us? Right here! [Referring to the Couples Focus Group].

Identity as a couple in recovery underscores an important developmental sequence in long-term recovery. Preliminary analysis of data at CCR on couples in various stages of addiction and recovery suggests that a relational focus throughout the stages of recovery is helpful, a position advocated by Covington and Surrey (Wellesley Centers for Women, Work in Progress, No. 91, 2000) and more recently, articulated in the Center for Substance Abuse Treatment publication, "Substance Abuse Treatment and the Family" (TIP No. 39, 2004). Individual work need not preempt appropriate concurrent relational therapies, even in early recovery.

An important treatment intervention in Shifting is asking the couple how alcoholism and recovery have affected their lives as a couple. Creating a dialogue around the concept of couple recovery and normalizing the difficulties and struggles couples experience through the stages of recovery provides a new way to explain and work with relational difficulties. It is important for therapists to acknowledge recovery histories and contextually place relationship changes and adaptation to recovery as significant factors in couple development. Prescribing exercises aimed at establishing or deepening a couple-family identity helps facilitate the important developmental process associated with shifting. Therapeutic work on establishing new rituals, finding mutually enjoyable activities or projects, and learning how to have fun together, help create a feeling of connection and belonging. Research couples often report problems with how to bond with their partners. Mary and Leo stated they used to feel close during "happy hour," when they would drink together and talk for several hours. When Mary got into recovery, she and Leo had to find new ways to connect and have fun together. Another therapy/research couple had never considered the notion of being a couple in recovery despite both being recovering alcoholics each with well over 10 years of continuous recovery and participation in AA. Helping them to identify, acknowledge, and normalize the difficulties of couple recovery provided a new language and way of understanding relationship problems. Incorporating couple recovery with their individual recoveries provided a bridge to connect recoveries and helped transcend the impasse they experienced in their relationship.

Intergenerational Reworking. The second component in the evolving couple restructuring in long-term recovery occurs through a deeper grasp of family dynamics in current and family of origin systems. Couples begin integrating a clearer understanding of the impact of their families of origin on their own development as individuals and in the couple relationship. The breakdown of denial about significant family of origin issues precedes, or in the very least, significantly impacts the couple's ability to more effectively deal with their own couple and family life functioning. Profound feelings of grief and loss emerge as the realities of family traumas are acknowledged, integrated, and appropriated.

Kyle speaks to the pervasive role of alcohol in his life his life. The meaning of alcohol, and ultimately the meaning of recovery and his relationships are seen in the context of his family history of alcoholism.

> Kyle: ...I can't ever imagine my father being in recovery. My father is the embodiment of alcoholism. He hasn't had a drink in a while, but he is alcoholism; that's him. I wouldn't know how to imagine him sober. Maybe it will come to me in a dream sometime. My mother is alcoholism. She doesn't drink but her whole life has been formed by his dependence. I can't imagine myself apart from alcoholism. It bursts into my life, and now recovery....

This key awareness filters into a deeper understanding of his individual recovery and on his recovery as a couple. Kyle saw in himself similar responses he experienced from his alcoholic father's relationship with him, with his siblings, and with Kyle's mother. Through a painful process of identification with his family's dysfunctional patterns, then with an awareness he could choose to operate differently, Kyle began integrating intergenerational work into his relationship with his wife and with his children.

> Kyle: I think, well, there's a certain point at which I hope to not contribute to that craziness anymore! That's the part I can change...

In the following excerpt Kyle speaks to a different understanding of what it means to love and be loved. His deepening understanding of the impact of his family of origin on his own individual and relational development allows him to see healthier ways of relating in his own family.

> Kyle: My father does love me, whatever love means to him. The byproduct of that love is drama. It was love that allowed him to beat the crap out of me, and tyrannize me, and terrorize me, and make everything so dramatic...I think that's what caught up with my early attempts to make sense of what love was...He loves me and I love him, so this must be love. When I got sober I think he thought something changed, and so did I. And I don't know what it is with us but I know that I can love other people, and probably him in another way, in that quieter way.

For many of the research couples alcohol has been the source of family connection. The couples often report that when they began recovery they experienced derision and rejection from their families. Acknowledging alcohol-related problems, or expressing feelings about those problems is often met with the painful re-traumatizing experience of feeling utter abandonment by parents and other family members, not an unusual feeling for someone growing up in an alcoholic family as the following quotations indicate.

> Betsy: It's just awful that need in families like that…you see that is the way it is in my family; it's very difficult to have anything going on if you're not drinking. So anybody going into that circle that doesn't drink won't fit…they try, but the alcohol is the conduit.
>
> Nan: I was just thinking when you were talking about your relationship with your father Betsy, it's definitely like alcohol being the umbilical cord to the family.
>
> Kyle: [Referring to his family and Nan's family] The drinking person is the healthy person. The nondrinking person is the unhealthy person; there is something wrong with us…I think the family that is still drinking continues to still have that sort of thing. In Nan's family I'm the one that has something wrong with him.
>
> Vic: I think that part of it too, is that part of the family that is still drinking resents others…Denial shows up in the family in the form of the alcoholic being viewed as normal rather than abnormal. To not drink is considered abnormal and sick.

Each of the participants in the focus group expressed awareness of the dysfunction in their family of origin. With varying degrees of insight, they often contrasted their healthier learned recovery behaviors with the denial they experience in the family of origin. The contrasts were especially striking in two areas: (a) acknowledgement of dysfunction, and (b) tolerating and expressing feelings of grief and sadness.

Over the course of the five year period Betsy's denial about her father's alcoholism eroded as she discussed family life and the role that alcohol had in her family. About one year into the group Betsy spoke about her father's drinking, she did not identify his drinking as a problem. In fact, this story was portrayed humorously.

Betsy: There are a whole lot of rituals. My father has a yellow glass; there are several different kinds of sets of glasses in their house. The yellow one is his and nobody else drinks out of yellow glasses. That's because he always mislaid his drink, and this way he could keep track of his drink. It's a family joke. A lot of our family jokes are around alcohol…

Three years later Betsy was struggling with feelings of grief and depression. She again referred to her parent's drinking, this time she expressed anger and betrayal.

Betsy: …that's the thing that makes me so angry…I've been working my ass off since I've been on my own to figure out what's wrong. Finally I got it, the alcohol! That was my moment of clarity, my God, alcohol…it's been really hard for me to acknowledge, to not deny my parent's drinking…

Kyle: You've got it now, it was always there.

Betsy: I know this is not malevolent on their part…it's just the way it was with them…but there is something I think connected to this anger that I have. Damn, I was ripped off…

Deep feelings of deprivation and dispossession followed Betsy's awareness that her parent's primary relationship had been with alcohol and not the children. Betsy tearfully expressed grief and anger in her statement "He forgot I was special." This powerful statement summarizes Betsy's feelings of abandonment, hurt, and betrayal.

Helping couples explore the impact of their family of origin on their own relational functioning forms the central therapeutic task in intergenerational reworking. Linking relationship functioning between family of origin and the current nuclear family structure delineates an individuating process from pathological family ties. Emotionally charged levels of grief and anger strongly correlated with increased awareness of unhealthy boundaries and the desire to break the chain of family dysfunction.

Focus group members all related to family injunctions against expressing anger, grief, or any negative feelings. While therapists need to evaluate for clinical depression, normalizing sadness given the reality of family life, helping partners support each other, and giving permission to break the family rule of silence, are all important therapeutic tasks in this component of couple recovery. A core developmental issue in couple recovery relates to the couple's ability to tolerate and integrate painful feelings, especially grief. The focus group couples acknowledged that tolerating psychological pain had taken a long time in recovery but they expressed relief at being able to feel their suffering rather than denying, fearing, or avoiding these negative emotions. The thought of coping with this awareness in early recovery was portrayed as overwhelming seemed unrealistic to the group.

Attending. The third component of ongoing couple recovery identifies improved couple functioning and increased emphasis on individual autonomy and growth. The couple now has a better skill set to manage affective experiences, communicate more clearly and honestly, and to experience deeper levels of trust and intimacy with each other. Most importantly, they are able to stay present to one another; fears of abandonment or rejection have lessened and the couple relationship has a resilience and fluidity to adapt to the emotional demands of life and of each other, marking a new developmental level in the couple relationship. Acceptance of each other, in marked contrast to performance orientation and perfectionism, increases the feeling of comfort, security, and acceptance in the relationship. Partner support and attunement reinforce growth. Fears of abandonment or rejection lessened and the couple relationship had resilience and fluidity to adapt to the emotional demands of life and of each other.

Previously, individual and couple recovery avenues appeared mutually exclusive. Now, an emphasis on couple and individual growth characterizes a developmental stage toward interdependency in context of an individuated self. Attending marks a couple's ability to manage concurrent recoveries, individual and couple, caring for self and caring for the partner.

> Leo: I think that what has happened is that I am much more accepting of Mary as she is. There is, I think, a major shift in my attitude for both giving and getting support. The changes have been so deep, so profound I could never go back.
>
> Nan: We have grown together as a couple a lot. Our sense of who we are has increased a lot. We're not as fearful of whether we can succeed. The world is not nearly as threatening as it was... And now we can grow separately, and in a way, closer.

Acknowledging ones own needs and needs of the partner means risking and talking about issues and feelings rather than holding on to them or denying them. Trust and willingness to risk open the way to communication so couples are better able to identify and express their feelings and concerns to one another without fear of rejection or humiliation. New psychological and spiritual resources are available to the couple allowing increased levels of relatedness so problems can be dealt with as they occur. Couples still struggle with many aspects of their relationship, but they now have a greater ability to tolerate conflict and work on issues together. For some, fears of abandonment and rejection are not as prominent and partners are more trusting while dealing with discord and difficulties.

As with Shifting and Intergenerational Reworking, couples vary in the degree of their ability to integrate the tasks of Attending into successful couple recovery. Some couples found it easier to give support than to receive support and vice versa. Comfort with closeness and intimacy differ as illustrated in the following exchange.

> Mary: Intimacy becomes something to deal with in sobriety; before, all that bugaboo stuff was covered for me by the alcohol, and now I have face: Who did I really marry?
> Betsy: That's what really happens for me…
> Mary: Am I willing to expose myself to this person that I have all these charged issues with, that I've only begun to understand?

In the past, attachments have been primarily with alcohol and through alcohol. Early recovery helps individuals to reconnect with themselves. In ongoing recovery, closeness with the significant other involves emotional vulnerability and requires a certain amount of trust and resilience in the relationship. Tolerating each other's emotional pain is one index of successful incorporation of Attending in the relationship.

> Mary: And we are in such a different place that I have the same feeling of joy and satisfaction that I'm in a good place with Leo's mother. I don't know if you know, Betsy, that Leo's mother is dying, I mean imminently. He's very needy now and able to show me how needy he is, and he is able to accept nurturing. He can…all of a sudden start to weep, and I'll just go over and hold on to him…It comes out of something new between us here…we are so much healthier, I don't have to be sick like Leo's mother.

Focus group couples identified continued difficulties and unresolved difficulties in their sexual relationship. Increased intimacy, trust, and communication did not translate into a more satisfying sexual relationship. An initial finding with subsequent research couples suggests sexuality as a significant problematic area. A better understanding of the factors and dynamics contributing to this difficulty are under study. The following comments were offered as part of only one of the two times sex was discussed at length over the five year period.

Kyle: I remember being in an AA meeting once and a woman asked, "Has anybody noticed any sexual problems in recovery?" Everyone started laughing and people said "Yes." She said rather angrily "I've been sober for six weeks and I would think that it would have been straightened out by now!" [Group laughter]; and then we really laughed [more group laughter]. But those are some of our issues and they're hard to talk about. Was sex different when you were drinking?

Betsy: Oh yeah, that's what sex is. That's what sex is with us, drinking. For me sex has always had to have alcohol or pot. Sex is a real problem for me.

Vic: Me too...

Betsy: And the thing with the sex is so puzzling to me because I feel like another gift of sobriety for me is that passion is awakened; I feel passionately about stuff. Before, I think I really needed the alcohol; that's where my passion was, or would get relieved, so it wasn't even mine. But I really feel now like I've got a self, I've got feelings, I can live, and I don't know where to go with it as far as our relationship is concerned...one of the reasons I focus on the time together is because I think that's the first step.

The rhythm of recovery in the Attending component of couple recovery flowed on strengths and self-validation rather than on what was wrong, or "character defects" as labeled in the 12-step programs. Meaningfulness and authenticity in relationships slowly replaces the fear and dishonesty that dominated interactions in the drinking and early recovery stages. Therapeutic and psychoeducational approaches in Attending address the following issues: (a) self-care and self-acceptance, (b) increased intimacy, (c) partner appreciation and support, (d) spirituality, and (e) sexuality.

A Nonlinear Perspective. CRDA conceptualizes alcoholism assessment and treatment from multiple and simultaneous levels of individual and couple dynamics with its numerous permutations in individual and couple recovery processes. Evidence of movement back and forth between stages unfolded in the monthly interactions and experiences shared by the members. Uneven levels of resolution not dependent on a specific progression gave evidence to the dynamic, interdependent nature of the relationship between Shifting, Intergenerational Reworking, and Attending.

Difficulties in one component of couple development, i.e., Shifting (forming a stronger couple identity), may well be affected by an unresolved area in another component like Intergenerational Reworking, where abandonment issues may trigger fear responses when getting closer. Conversely, closer emotional ties with the spouse in Shifting and Attending may be a source of healing for relational wounds from the family of origin. The specific variables in each area and how they interact with each other will differ greatly between couples, as does the degree of resolution in the components. CRDA theory proposes that recovery remains an ongoing developmental process impacted by the interactivity of these three areas of couple development.

CONCLUSION

Studies on addiction and the family suggest the importance of a relational perspective in the overall conceptualization of recovery processes. "Couple recovery" and the reciprocal relationship between individual and relational dynamics, more fully account for the complexity of addiction/recovery processes and the need for multiple levels of intervention in alcoholism treatment, a notion challenging current assumptions that individual and family recoveries are mutually exclusive.

Prevailing research and treatment paradigms emphasize outcome measures to the number of days the alcoholic remains abstinent, unfortunately disregarding the couple-family system. Longitudinal research on treatment modalities incorporating relationally- and individually-oriented approaches in an overall conceptualization of recovery processes supports the need for increased understanding of the reciprocal nature of the dynamics between the alcoholic and the couple relationship throughout phases of addiction and recovery. Future research aimed at tailoring recoveries specifically to the transitions and developmental needs of the individuals and couple relationship offers a new direction in alcoholism treatment.

CRDA, an evolving theory of long-term couple recovery, delineates three discrete, yet interrelated components of couple development: Shifting, Intergenerational Reworking, and Attending. Nonlinear, interactive dynamics between these components constitute the overall direction of couple recovery.

REFERENCES

Bertalanffy, L. von. (1969). *General systems theory.* New York: George Braziller.

Brown, S. (1985). *Treating the alcoholic.* New York: John Wiley & Sons.

Brown, S., & Lewis, V. (1995). The alcoholic family: A developmental model of recovery. In S. Brown (Ed.), *Treating Alcoholism* (pp. 279-315). San Francisco: Jossey-Bass Publishers.

Brown, S., & Lewis, V. M. (1999). *The alcoholic family in recovery: A developmental model.* New York: Guilford.

Center for Substance Abuse Treatment. (2004). *Substance abuse treatment and family therapy, treatment Improvement protocol Series, No. 39.* (DHHS Publication No. SMA 04-3957, TIP). Rockville, MD. Substance Abuse and Mental Health Services Administration.

Edwards, M. E., & Steinglass, P. (1995). Family therapy treatment outcomes for alcoholism. *Journal of Marital and Family Therapy, 21*(4), 475-509.

Fichter, M. M., Glynn, S. M., Weyerer, S., & Liberman, R. P. (1997). Family climate and expressed emotion in the course of alcoholism. *Family Process, 36*(2), 202-221.

Gilgun, J. F., Daly, K., & Handle, G. (1992). *Qualitative methods in family research.* Newbury Park: Sage Publications.

Glaser, B. G., & Strauss, A. L. (1967). *The discovery of grounded theory: Strategies for qualitative research.* New York: Aldine De Gruyer.

Heath, A. W., and Stanton, M. D. (1998). Family-based treatment. In R. J. Frances, & S. I. Miller (Eds.), *Clinical textbook of addictive disorders* (2nd ed., pp. 496-520). New York: Guilford Press.

Humphreys, K., Moos, R. H., & Cohen, C. (1997). Social and community resources and long-term recovery from treated and untreated alcoholism. *Journal of Studies on Alcohol, 58*(3), 231-238.

Jacob, T. (1992). Family studies of alcoholism. *Journal of Family Psychology, 5*(3 & 4), 319-338.

McCrady, B. S. (1990). The marital relationship and alcoholism treatment. In R. I. Collins, K. E. Leonard, & J. S. Searles (Eds.), *Alcohol and the family* (pp.338-353). New York: Guilford Press.

McCrady, B. S., & Epstein, E. E. (1995). Directions for research on alcoholic relationships: Marital- and individual-based models of heterogeneity. *Psychology of Addictive Behaviors, 9*(3), 157-166.

Moos, R. H., & Moos, B. S. (1984). The process of recovery from alcoholism: Comparing functioning in families of alcoholics and matched control families. *Journal of studies on Alcoholism, 45*(2), 111-118.

Navarra, R. J. (2002). Couples in recovery from alcoholism: Long-term and developmental processes (Doctoral dissertation, California Institute of Integral Studies, 2002). *Dissertation Abstracts International, 63-02B*, 3042888.

Navarra, R. J. (2003, Summer). Treating couples in recovery from alcoholism. *The AAMFT-CA Division News, 11*, 1-3.

Navarra, R. J. (2003, Fall). Treating couples in recovery from alcoholism: Part 2. *The AAMFT-CA Division News, 12*, 1-3.

O'Farrell, T. J. (1992). Families and alcohol problems: An overview of treatment research. *Journal of Family Psychology, 5*(3 & 4), 339-359.

O'Farrell, T. J., Hooley, J., Fals-Stewart, W., & Cutter, H. S. G. (1998). Expressed emotion and relapse in alcoholic patients. *Journal of Consulting and Clinical Psychology, 66*(5), 744-752.

Preli, R., Protinsky, H., & Cross, L. (1990). Alcoholism and family structure. *Family Therapy,17*(1), 1-7.

Rotunda, R. J., Scherer, D. G., & Imm, P. S. (1995). Family systems and alcohol misuse: Research on the effects of alcoholism on family functioning and effective family interventions. *Professional Psychology: Research and Practice, 26*(1), 95-104.

Stanton, M. D., & Shadish, W.R. (1997). Outcome, attrition, and family-couples treatment for drug abuse: A meta-analysis and review of the controlled, comparative studies. *Psychological Bulletin, 122*(2), 170-191.

Steinglass, P. (1976). Experimenting with family treatment approaches to alcoholism, 1950-1975: A review. *Family Process, 15*(1), 97-123.

Steinglass, P. (1985). Family systems approaches to alcoholism. *Journal of Substance Abuse, 2*, 161-167.

Steinglass, P., Bennett, L. A., Wolin, S. J., & Reiss, D. (1987). *The alcoholic family.* New York: Basic Books.

Steinglass, P., Tislenko, L., Reiss, D. (1985). Stability/instability in the alcoholic marriage: The interrelationships between course of alcoholism, family process, and marital outcome. *Family Process, 23*(3), 365-376.

Usher, M. L., Jay, J., & Glass, D. R. (1982). Family therapy as a treatment modality for alcoholism. *Journal of Studies on Alcohol, 43*(9), 927-938.

Wellesley Centers for Women, (2000). *The relational model of women's psychological development: Implications for substance abuse* (Work in Progress, No. 91). Wellesley: Covington, S. S., & Surrey, J. L.

Winters, J., Fals-Stewart, W., O'Farrell, T. J., Birchler, G. R., & Kelley, M. L. (2000). Behavioral couples therapy for female substance-abusing patients: Effects on substance use and relationship adjustment. *Journal of Consulting and Clinical Psychology, 70*(2), 344-355.

doi:10.1300/J020v25n01_06

Coping Strategies for the Stages
of Family Recovery

Virginia Lewis, PhD
Lois Allen-Byrd, PhD

SUMMARY. This paper introduces and briefly discusses the concept of family recovery and the research that identified the four stages of recovery. The main focus, however, is to discuss the role of the therapist in treating families in recovery; including working with children; and to identify and discuss the different requirements, tasks, and treatment strategies associated with each stage. Therapists can play a vital role in two main ways when working with alcoholic families: (1) to assist the family in entering into the recovery process and (2) to help them maintain recovery. To do this effectively, therapists must first understand the characteristics of family recovery–it is only then that can they provide coping strategies for the recovering alcoholic, co-alcoholic, and children. For example, the therapist begins with a concrete, active, practical approach (transition and early recovery stages) and moves into a more psychodynamic, inter-active, approach (ongoing recovery stage) as exemplified in the coping strategies and ideas presented in the paper. However, it is important to remember that recovery is a process that does not have demarcations for

Virginia Lewis is Co-Founder and Co-Director of the Family Recovery Project, Mental Research Institute (MRI), Palo Alto, California.

Lois Allen-Byrd is affiliated with the Mental Research Institute (MRI), Palo Alto, California.

Address correspondence to: Virginia Lewis, PhD, Mental Research Institute (MRI), 555 Middlefield Rd., Palo Alto, CA 94301 (E-mail: famrec@ix.netcom.com).

[Haworth co-indexing entry note]: "Coping Strategies for the Stages of Family Recovery." Lewis, Virginia, and Lois Allen-Byrd. Co-published simultaneously in *Alcoholism Treatment Quarterly* (The Haworth Press, Inc.) Vol. 25, No. 1/2, 2007, pp. 105-124; and: *Familial Responses to Alcohol Problems* (ed: Judith L. Fischer, Miriam Mulsow, and Alan W. Korinek) The Haworth Press, Inc., 2007, pp. 105-124. Single or multiple copies of this article are available for a fee from The Haworth Document Delivery Service [1-800-HAWORTH, 9:00 a.m. - 5:00 p.m. (EST). E-mail address: docdelivery@haworthpress.com].

Available online at http://atq.haworthpress.com
doi:10.1300/J020v25n01_07

the beginning and ending of each stage. Rather, recovery is fluid with an ebb and flow of individual and family dynamics and interactions. doi:10.1300/J020v25n01_07 *[Article copies available for a fee from The Haworth Document Delivery Service: 1-800-HAWORTH. E-mail address: <docdelivery@haworthpress.com> Website: <http://www.HaworthPress.com> © 2007 by The Haworth Press, Inc. All rights reserved.]*

KEYWORDS. Family recovery, stages of recovery, treatment and coping strategies by stages

INTRODUCTION

It is a widely held belief that once an alcoholic stops drinking, life for all family members will become "normal." In actuality, however, abstinence marks the beginning of a journey that is profoundly difficult for all family members. Without guidance, support, and knowledge of the recovery process, most people will relapse. As such, it is incumbent upon alcoholics and co-alcoholics to utilize external resources (therapists, 12-step programs, and sponsors) to maintain their sobriety and to facilitate their progress through the stages of recovery. It is crucial for therapists who are working with clients in the active process of maintaining sobriety to understand the recovery process. That said, the purpose of this paper is twofold. The first is to briefly describe the four stages of recovery as experienced by alcoholics and co-alcoholics. The second is to provide therapists with coping and therapeutic strategies associated with each stage of family recovery. It is hoped that with the increased knowledge of what families experience as they move through recovery, therapists will be able to understand why certain strategies are recommended at particular times, and to help them create stage-appropriate coping skills for their clients.

BACKGROUND

In 1989, Drs. Stephanie Brown and Virginia Lewis developed the Family Recovery Project–the primary intent of which was to study the recovery processes in the alcoholic family when one or both spouses stopped drinking. To date, this exploratory research remains the only one that studies the recovery of the family (as compared to that of the individual).

The essential two-part question posed by the Project Co-Directors was: What is the normal process of recovery in the alcoholic family, and does it change with time? To answer these questions, a cross-sectional design was used to look at fifty-two families in varying lengths of recovery (two months to eighteen years). Each family participated in a three-hour videotaped interview and a battery of paper and pencil tests to assess individual, couple, and family functioning. (Details of the methodology and family measures can be found in Brown & Lewis, 1995, 1999.)

Family Recovery Model

In order to capture the complexity of family recovery, two dimensions–time and domain–were required. Time is noted by four developmental stages of recovery: drinking, transition, early recovery, and ongoing recovery. Domain is the perspective used to assess an aspect of the family. The three domains are: the environment (the atmosphere in which the family functions), the system (how the family functions, e.g., roles, rules, and routines), and the individual (individual behavioral patterns, cognitions, and emotions). The Family Recovery Model allows for the identification of themes, dynamics, and events that change with time and within different domains.

Family Recovery Stages

Families have taught us that there are identifiable themes and tasks associated with each stage of recovery. The following are brief descriptions of the four stages.

Drinking stage. Alcohol organizes both the family system and each member during this stage. On an individual level, the alcoholic's primary relationship is with alcohol, while the spouse's central focus is in reaction to the alcoholic. The family system is governed by rules and regulatory processes that allow for the domination of alcohol to be maintained. The environment can be tense and hostile, or it can be experienced more subtly through the constriction and restriction of perceptions, behaviors, and emotions (a "psychological straight jacket" of sorts).

Transition stage. In this stage, the individual alcoholic is moving from drinking to abstinence. As drinking becomes increasingly out of control, the alcoholic "hits bottom" and stops drinking. If both spouses go into a recovery, the family system also hits bottom. This spiraling-out-of-control is characterized by unpredictability; broken promises; increased family and marital distress, even violence. The shift from drinking to sobriety in this stage is filled with confusion, turmoil, and the mixed pain of relief from drinking and terror of what is next. According to our research families, the beginning of the recovery process is the most difficult, if not the most traumatic time, as the bottom has dropped out and nothing works at the individual or systemic domains.

Early recovery stage. Adults in early recovery learn new ways to handle urges to drink and to rescue. They begin to learn self-responsibility and new skills to create a healthier life at the behavioral level, e.g., making sure children are attended to, meals are put on the table, and practical routines established. Through sponsors and/or therapists, they learn not to lean on the marriage to solve their problems or to have their needs met. Instead, their task is to find new approaches to take care of their own needs. This period can last from three to five years and is a time to reconstruct the family system slowly, and on the practical and structural levels (e.g., new roles, rules, and routines).

Ongoing recovery stage. Ongoing recovery is a time of refining and fine tuning the self, the system, and relationships as the recovery processes for individuals in the family are becoming internalized and stabilized. The home environment begins to feel safe, secure, and pleasant, and the family system is fundamentally working at the functional and structural levels (e.g., daily routines have been established and adjusted as needed, the flow of family life works more effectively). If problems arise, there is increasing confidence that family members can attend to and resolve them. For example, urges to drink or sacrificially caretake are handled by established behavioral patterns and/or cognitive processes. (See Brown, Lewis, & Liotta, 2000; Brown & Lewis, 1999; Brown & Lewis, 1995 for a detailed description of the family recovery model.)

It should be noted that there are no clear indicators that mark the ending of one stage and the beginning of the next. Recovery *is a process* that is at times linear (developmentally) and at other times, circular (2 different components interacting thus creating a dynamic process).

However, there are specific tasks and assessment criteria that can be used to identify which stage the individual and/or family is in. For example, when in the abstinence phase of Transition, the impulses to drink and to rescue are dominant and are contained by a practical concrete focus on attending 12-step meetings, developing a new identity, and new beliefs. Early Recovery denotes less dominance of impulses, extending the knowledge and practice of recovery beliefs, and a deepening attachment and commitment to AA/AlAnon and sobriety. As impulsivity decreases and attachment to external sources are established, the overt dependency needs decrease and the individual moves into Ongoing Recovery. In this stage, recovery is maintained, and identity, beliefs, and attachments are becoming internalized. (The qualitative aspects found in each stage are detailed in Chapter 6 and Figure 6.1 in *The Alcoholic Family in Recovery* (1999).)

Treatment Emphasis by Stages

Each recovery stage has its own emphasis/focus which translates into different treatment approaches which, in turn, impact the five areas of human experiences: behavioral, cognitive, emotional, social/interpersonal, and spiritual. These five areas are the building blocks for separation and individuation from the alcoholic family dynamics, the development of a healthier family system, and future healthy attachments to family members and others. The focus for each of the three stages of recovery is as follows:

> *Transition*: In this stage the approach is practical and pragmatic with an emphasis on the behavioral level, e.g., how to handle daily life, addictive urges, be parents, go to meetings, and work with sponsors and therapists.
> *Early Recovery*: The approach in this stage continues to be practical and behavioral. However, there is significant learning that sets the foundation for emotional, cognitive, social, and spiritual growth. In addition, a new family system, organized around recovery, is becoming established. Individuals in the family are acquiring sober identities, learning self-responsibility, and increasing parenting skills.
> *Ongoing Recovery*: In this stage the approach is more psychodynamic and reflective. Insight is used to facilitate change within oneself and in relation to others. Alcoholics and co-alcoholics are learning to become a couple again in healthy ways. They are hearing and tolerating the pain that their children experienced during the drinking years, and internalizing the structures and coping mechanisms needed to maintain recovery.

Each stage of recovery, with its corresponding approaches, is crucial to maintaining sobriety, growth, and healthy relationships. As stated earlier, what is important to remember is that recovery is a process and although each stage has its own tasks and themes, there are no rigid do's and don'ts. For example, insight can occur in the Transition Stage, and practical and behavioral changes can take place in the Ongoing Recovery Stage, and throughout life. The stages are ways of understanding and grasping time and the key factors and approaches necessary to increase the potential for maintaining recovery.

EXPERIENTIAL DESCRIPTION OF EACH STAGE

The following experiential descriptions and subsequent coping strategies are based on anecdotal material obtained from analyzing hundreds of hours of videotapes of the family interviews. (The interview questions can be found in Appendix A in *The Alcoholic Family in Recovery* (Brown & Lewis, 1999) and for specific factors related to successful family recovery, please refer to *Understanding Successful Recovery: Two Models* (Lewis, Allen-Byrd, & Rouhbakhsh, 2004).)

Transition Recovery Stage

The Transition Recovery Stage is the part of the journey that is like riding a never-ending roller coaster that is out of control. At times it feels as if the recovering person is struggling uphill every inch of the way only to find him or herself plummeting back down to earth. He/she does not recognize or understand any of the signposts or scenery flashing by and may think, "Am I going crazy?," "I can't make it," "It's too hard," "Drinking wasn't so bad," or "Maybe I'm not an alcoholic/ co-alcoholic." It is important for the therapist to realize and convey to the alcoholic that all of this is normal for this stage and that things will improve.

Early Recovery Stage

One day the realization comes that the roller coaster experience has been replaced with a train ride. Although there are hills and valleys, this journey seems to be equipped with pull cords for brakes and stops. It feels exciting and scary at the same time.

During this stage, the train stops at many stations to allow for taking in and letting go. New experiences and learning abound. Recovering individuals are acquiring new ways to be in the world and are discarding excess baggage. Faith is turning into trust and confidence. Common comments are: "Maybe I can," "Sobriety is possible," "I don't know the answer now, but that's OK, I might in the future."

Ongoing Recovery Stage

The recovery ride is more stable in this stage. Strategies for handling impulses, difficult emotions, and diffusing potential crises are becoming internalized. There is a large and varied repertoire of coping skills available that allows for choices, flexible thinking, and problem solving.

COPING STRATEGIES BY STAGES

The following section offers some general coping strategies to help families in each of the three stages. These strategies are appropriate for alcoholics and co-alcoholics alike unless otherwise noted.

Transition Recovery Coping Strategies

The transition stage is marked by overwhelming cravings, impulses (to drink or to rescue), and a swirl of emotions. In order to cope more effectively with these emerging feelings and impulses, they need to be turned into an action. In other words, affective regulation is obtained by behavioral action (as will be discussed in the next section). It is important for therapists to be aware of and to tell their clients that this stage requires dependency–dependency upon external resources such as sponsors, meetings, and therapists. It is crucial that therapists normalize this stage by supporting and teaching the need to learn, identify, and use healthy outside resources. (Participants in the Family Recovery Project who were successful in maintaining recovery learned to utilize outside resources while internal structures were being slowly developed (Brown & Lewis, 1999; Lewis, Allen-Byrd, & Rouhbakhsh, 2004).)

Therapists who are inexperienced and working with recovering couples and/or families may consider consultation with an experienced therapist in this field. Therapists need to be active, to be supportive of healthy dependency, to define and develop with the couple guidelines in seeking assistance outside the office sessions. Most of the early recovery years involve handling impulses to use/rescue and to regulate the emotional turmoil. Therapy, in conjunction with the clients' participation in 12-step programs, helps clients navigate those early years successfully.

Transition Coping Strategy Ideas

The following are some suggestions that therapists can give to their clients to help them through the frequently tumultuous Transition Stage.

1. Write a list of actions to be used when you experience an impulse or emotion. These actions can be developed with a sponsor and/or therapist and/or Old Timer in a 12-step program. Keep this list with you at all times. These action items help contain emotional fluctuations and shift the focus from acting out to developing recovery tools. For example, write the following strategies on a 3 × 5 card:

    (a) Call sponsor. Phone number: _____
    (b) Call "safe friends" Name: _____Phone Number: _____
    (c) Create a mantra to help you over the rough moments. Pick one that has meaning to you, e.g., "This will pass," "I can do it," "Turn it over," "Hold on until I get to a meeting," "It's like labor pain and I made it," etc.
    (d) List of 12-step meetings–times and places.
    (e) Listen to a tape by your therapist talking to you soothingly.
    (f) Use a small object given to you by your therapist, safe friend, and/or sponsor and hold it in your hand for anchoring and feeling safe.

2. Think of soothing places to visit, and add them to the 3 × 5 list. For example, see the sunset; hear the ocean; walk along a specific beach/lake/river/park, etc; stroll through a favorite store (if you are not a spendaholic); florist, etc.
3. Breathe. This is perhaps the best overall coping mechanism. Breathe deeply and slowly. By doing so you cannot remain anxious/ fearful.
4. Take up a physical activity that is easily accessible. For example: jogging, power walking, pushups, yoga, shooting baskets, biking, (and other frequented places like a gym), etc.
5. For the alcoholic, develop new routes to and from work, the gym, in order to bypass a favorite drinking place.
6. For the co-alcoholic, write down specific co-alcoholic behaviors on one side of the paper and specific actions to substitute on the other side. For example:

Co-Alcoholic Behavior	*Action*
Checking on/Calling spouse at work.	Call sponsor/therapist, even if it is only to leave a message on the answering machine.
Worrying spouse is drinking. Staying up until spouse comes home.	Write worry down and burn it. Mantra: "I cannot control another, only myself."
	Listen to soothing tapes, sleep in another room, or engage in a pleasurable hobby.

7. Find and keep a copy of a favorite passage from scriptures, a poem, or a book. Read it deeply and fully.
8. Write down how alcohol has impacted your life. Make a list from it to remind you during moments of denial and confusion. For example, when the question arises, "Am I really an alcoholic/co-alcoholic?" you can respond with:

I am an alcoholic because:

(a) I went to work/drove in blackouts.
(b) I had fights with my spouse that I do not remember.
(c) I lost jobs or had DUIs or car accidents due to drinking.
(d) My spouse said he/she would leave me if I drank again.
(e) I lost the respect of my children.
(f) I watched my child begin his/her career in drinking/drugs, etc.

I am a co-alcoholic because:

(a) My entire focus became my drinking spouse.
(b) I made continued excuses for his/her behaviors.
(c) I "tiptoed" around my spouse to minimize fights/abuse.
(d) I told the children to not "rock the boat."
(e) I woke up one day too tired/depressed to go on this way.
(f) I took on extra work to bail out the family from continued financial crisis.

(g) I lost myself along the way.
(h) I felt like I was going crazy.

(Adapted from Brown, Lewis, & Liotta, 2002)

Early Recovery Coping Strategies

This stage is highlighted by the absence of alcohol, detachment from enmeshed relationships, a new identity formation, working the steps, individual growth, and developing solid external support. Of particular importance is detachment–given its association with letting go of the bottle and/or one's spouse. For example, how one related to his or her spouse or to alcohol was at the extreme expense of one's self and healthy development which ultimately resulted in unhealthy self-sacrifice.

One of the hallmarks of this stage is the awareness that the cravings and impulses have decreased. The energy, concentration, and action required to manage these gripping experiences are now freer to acquire a wealth of new learning. With the advent of detachment, energy can be refocused on developing a new recovery identity and a stronger sense of self. Thus, this stage becomes a time of mental, emotional, and social growth and expression. While the focus remains on the individual and not the couple, the emphasis at the family level is on developing parental responsibilities and slowly acquiring healthier parenting skills.

Early Recovery Coping Strategy Ideas

The following are coping strategies that can be used for developing and maintaining detachment, acquiring self-responsibility and new recovery identities, and developing healthy parenting skills. Again, these are skills that therapists can teach family members. In fact, therapists can present these ideas to clients in the following written format:

1. When your attention is on alcohol and/or your partner, ask yourself, "What do I need to do for myself at this moment?" "What does this outside focus mean for me?" Check for HALTS (if you are Hungry, Angry, Lonely, Tired, Sick, or Stressed).
2. If in doubt about what to do (this is particularly confusing when it involves your partner), call your sponsor, therapist, and/or reach out to external support for suggestions.
3. When the *fear of drinking* comes up either for yourself and/or your partner, check to see if it is signaling danger signs. For example,

the alcoholic decides to visit an old drinking buddy or goes by the favorite bar; the co-alcoholic backslides in an attempt to again control over the alcoholic or begins to reinvest energies and focus on the alcoholic.

The response to any of the above is to take ACTION (See Transition Coping Strategy Ideas).

4. An area of grave difficulty for the recovering alcoholic is when his or her partner continues drinking and/or is uninvolved in the recovery process. The marital system remains alcoholic thus all of the old ways of relating, coping, problem solving, and communicating are defensive, resistant to change, chronically tense, and perhaps even violent. At times it feels like you are going crazy which is not surprising since you are living two diametrically opposite lifestyles (sobriety at the individual level vs. alcoholic at the family system level). In this situation, the main coping strategy is to focus on maintaining sobriety—*it is the number one priority*. This can be accomplished through:

    (a) Stabilizing alcoholic/co-alcoholic identity and acceptance of loss of control.
    (b) Attending 12-step meetings and working the steps.
    (c) Developing a strong working relationship with sponsor.
    (d) Having program friends to whom you can relate honestly.
    (e) Working with a therapist who understands family recovery; in particular, the impact of the non-recovery spouse on sobriety.

    In time, your spouse may perceive what he or she is missing in life and the marriage, and become involved in recovery. Or, as recovery becomes stronger over time, decide not to stay in the marriage as the price is too high. Remember to be patient as recovery is one step at a time and decisions do not need to be made quickly.
5. In this stage, the family focus is on parenting responsibilities and skill building. Marital issues and more emotionally laden family issues are set aside for later work. This separation of focus can be very difficult to accomplish and maintain. Too much pain, resentment, and rage can interrupt and interfere with responsible parenting.

Outside help is crucial to navigate these muddy and choppy waters. For example:

(a) Find an experienced family therapist who will focus on practical and basic parenting skill building and practical suggestions. The focus is on clear, direct, practical how-to's for each person, such as:

    (1) Task assignments. for a more effective home life
    (2) Building routines for the children.
    (3) Finding safe friends/family members as resources for the children.
    (4) Developing clear communication skills between the parents to facilitate parenting duties.

(b) Ask friends you respect in 12-step programs who have more experience in recovery than you about parenting ideas and suggestions they found helpful.

(c) Read books on parenting that the bookstore, friends, librarian recommend.

(d) When it gets tough, pause and remember the importance of your children. It is not about you and your spouse, but the kids. Also, remember to take breaks and to self-care and to breathe. You will have years of being a parent and time to develop this relationship.

(Adapted from Brown, Lewis, & Liotta, 2002)

Ongoing Recovery Coping Strategies

This stage of the recovery journey is a time of refining individual growth and sobriety. One's identity as an alcoholic/co-alcoholic and abstinent behaviors are now stabilized. External behavioral controls and coping skills are more internalized so one is freer to reflect and analyze impulses, dynamics, interactive patterns, and emotions. These internal mechanisms now replace the need for direct action. It is safe to redirect the focus on couple and family issues that were too painful to work with in the past. It is the time to work through the consequences of alcoholism and co-alcoholism to oneself and family.

The joy and relative smoothness of this stage is found in couples when both spouses are in recovery. This means that each individual, as well as the marital and family systems, are changing and growing. There is a profound significance on the type and quality of family recovery when both spouses are in recovery compared to when only the alcoholic spouse is in recovery (Lewis & Allen-Byrd, 2001). For example, when only one partner is in recovery, the marital/family system remains defensive, disjointed by frequent crisis-type interruptions and chronic underlying tensions.

However, when both spouses are in recovery, this stage is highlighted by stability, integration, deepening of awareness, insights, spirituality, and a growing ability of balancing of the I and We. These growing strengths are/were hard-earned.

Alcoholism and sobriety are always present, even in this stage, but at a different level (it is one of acceptance and becomes a living part of one's life). The traumatic experiences and crises related to drinking are now in the past which allows the consequences of earlier behaviors to be addressed without threatening sobriety. Normal family developmental issues and crises (marriage, births, illness, deaths) occur in the context of healthier individual and couple coping skills.

Some of the issues that occur during this stage, such as anger, intimacy, and unresolved issues with the children, can now be appropriately addressed. This requires that all who are involved are able to accept self-evaluation, self-responsibility, and a willingness to struggle through the difficult times. It is expected that by now, there has been separation and individuation by the family members (individual self-growth) and separation from the alcoholic enmeshed system that will allow healthier responses to difficult issues arising from the active alcoholic past.

Ongoing Recovery Coping Strategy Ideas

In this stage, couple and/or family therapy is quite helpful. It is a time to work through past intense feelings, develop intimacy, and resolve the pain and hurt that children experienced during the drinking period. The following are suggestions for therapists to focus on and can be presented to clients in the following manner:

1. Use of self-reflection to deal with unpleasant emotions:

    (a) Name the feelings.
    (b) Identify where the feelings come from.
    (c) Decide what to do with the feelings (i.e., do they need action now or just acknowledgement?)

2. Identify if an issue is an individual, couple, or family one:

   (a) What, if anything, needs to be done.
   (b) What is my part in it.
   (c) When to bring up this issue.
   (d) What my needs are and how to meet them.

3. Remember that both life and recovery are processes which provide a framework of patience, hope, and an ease on self and others.
4. When feeling that progress is not being made, write down the changes that have made over the years. You may be surprised as progress is subtle in this stage and may even go unnoticed.
5. Anger issues come from the difficulties of separating the old shame/blame dynamics from a healthy expression of anger. When anger occurs, it can feel like an emotional relapse. The following are coping strategy suggestions:

   (a) Identify what you are angry about. Was it triggered by a past or present event?
   (b) Decide how to handle the anger (journal writing, telling the person, telling your sponsor).
   (c) Consider letting the anger go. How important is it? If you let it go, will it lead to resentment?
   (d) Own the anger as it is about feelings. For example, "I was angry and disappointed when you did not keep your promise to me. I want to talk this through with you as it is important to me."

6. There is a fear of intimacy in this stage which stems from reconnecting/joining with another as it may "feel" like alcoholic enmeshment. The task at this stage is to develop a balance between I (individuality) and We (intimacy/bonding).
   The following are suggestions for coping strategies:

   (a) Is this closeness at anyone's expense?
   (b) Is this closeness a need or a want? Needs, i.e., neediness, can come from unconscious places which can be slippery. Wants involve more conscious decision-making.
   (c) Is the closeness causing problems, e.g., clinginess, outbursts, triggering abandonment feelings?

(d) Do both of you feel enriched by the intimate moment?

(e) If difficulties arise, teach separation and self-care. Later, reflect on what happened.

7. This stage is the time to deal with the problems that occurred for the children during the drinking years.

(Adapted from Brown, Lewis, & Liotta, 2002)

EXAMPLE OF A TRANSITIONAL RECOVERY STAGE STRATEGY

The following is a detailed example of a coping strategy used in the Transitional stage. It is a specific approach that therapists can use with clients who are struggling with recovery. Note how the emphasis in on practical, action-oriented problem solving which is a "tool" for learning how to avert potential crises.

With the help of the recovering couple/family, the therapist identifies an area that is problematic and asks specific questions that can be answered in concrete, practical/behavioral ways. For example, suppose the co-alcoholic has the thought, "I worry a lot that my spouse will go back to drinking." The therapist can propose questions to be addressed regarding the worry and work with the clients to develop some possible responses. The following is an example of potential questions and answers.

1. *What specifically needs to change?*

   (a) My worry.

2. *How will you know it has changed?*

   (a) My thinking will not be consumed by worry.
   (b) I will not nag or ask my spouse how he/she is feeling.
   (c) I will not monitor his/her actions to see if he/she is drinking.
   (d) My stomach won't be in knots.
   (e) I will be able to enjoy activities that used to interest me.

3. *What is your part in it and what can you do to change?*

   (a) To not nag, "snoop," etc.
   (b) To not sound accusatory when talking.

4. *Who else can you ask for ideas, suggestions, or help on this concern?*

    (a) My AlAnon sponsor, AlAnon meetings
    (b) My friend who has "been there, changed that."

5. *What aspect is in your power to change and what is not?*

    (a) I can learn to stop the worry.
    (b) I cannot control my spouse's sobriety.

6. *What is the behavioral plan?*

    (a) When I find myself worrying I will call my therapist, sponsor, or friend.
    (b) I will shift my focus of worry to an action (go for drink of water, pull weeds, write down the worry and put it in a box, go for a run, pull a rubber band on wrist and say "Stop!").
    (c) I can keep a log or record of times in day/week that I stopped the worry, the nagging, the snooping, etc. I can keep a weekly growth chart that records the number of times that I stopped behaviors that were related to worry and/or lessened the worry.
    (d) I can share my progress/relapse with my sponsor and/or informed (safe) friends.
    (e) Review with my therapist my behavioral plans frequently to reinforce the new learning and continue the resolution of the problem.

The above is an example of how therapists can provide therapeutic exercises that create recovery and coping skills that foster the maintenance of sobriety. Such exercises can be developed for each stage and modified as needed for each family.

CHILDREN'S ISSUES

There is a wealth of information on the impact of alcoholism on children. We know that children are victims of alcoholic families and that their development is sacrificed to maintain the denial required for the alcoholism to continue (Brown, Lewis, & Liotta, 2002; Brown & Lewis,

1999). What is not well known is that recovery is traumatic for children. While this appears surprising and contrary to our culture's belief that abstinence is the endpoint (e.g., once the alcoholic quits drinking, family life will somehow automatically and magically become "normal"), in reality, children are typically ignored during the recovery process. In fact, the one regret that parents expressed repeatedly in our research was how they "forgot" their children during the early years of recovery. For example, parents are attending meetings, going to therapy, or talking to "strangers" (e.g., sponsors) about how they are struggling with not drinking or how they are changing.

The following vignette briefly describes a fairly common scenario for a child in an alcoholic family, as well as provides suggestions for possible coping strategies to deal with the issues that are raised by the changing family dynamics. In this family, one child, Kayla, was designated as the caretaker of the alcoholic parent, thus eliciting the other parent's gratitude for Kayla's assistance. Kayla helped make household decisions on a daily basis and had special privileges that the other children did not. Now that the family is in recovery, Kayla is told that her previous role of caretaker no longer exists, nor is even desired, as the family no longer functions as it once did. Instead, as the alcoholic parent takes on more responsibilities, power is taken away from Kayla leaving her feeling, among other things, confused and angry. Kayla now has no anchor, familiar structure, or understanding of how to be in this recovering family and she may begin to act out at one extreme or withdraw at the other end.

This is a typical scenario for all family members, as in the initial period of family recovery, the roles, rules, routines, and ways of communicating and interacting begin to collapse which then creates a vacuum in the family system. Anger, resentments, and fear are common responses by children such as Kayla during the early recovery years and they frequently begin to act out during these stages in an attempt to regain control and/or express their feelings.

Child Focused Coping Strategies

The therapist can be instrumental in helping children make the transition into the earlier years of recovery by providing a safe place for them to express their fears, confusions, and anger; by providing age-appropriate explanations of what recovery is; and by normalizing the recovery process. The following are some ideas for the therapist to consider when working with issues such as those described above.

1. Work with the adults on parenting skills.
2. Have the parents explain alcoholism and recovery in terms that children can understand, i.e., make it age appropriate.
3. If the parents are too overwhelmed in early recovery, make sure the children have safe adults with whom they can visit and talk.
4. Provide the opportunity for children to become involved in AlAnon, AlaKid, AlaTot.
5. Let children know they are not responsible for their parent's alcoholism, recovery, or relapse.
6. While a new family system is evolving, help parents develop some structure in the family to help children feel secure. For example, dinner will always be provided and served at a specific time.
7. Encourage parents to ask for help when they encounter parent-child problems. Obtaining external assistance provides parents with new parental coping skills, more options in problem solving, and a protection from relapsing into past alcoholic black or white thinking and responses.
8. Children may be referred for individual therapy to help them in finding their way into a newly emerging family structure. Focus would be on assisting them in defining their own individuality and in working through role changes, resentments, and confusion.

Typically in the Ongoing Stage of Recovery, children will begin to trust their parents and the recovery process as they experience their parents' increasing predictability, responsibility, and willingness to hear and respond to them in healthier ways. This is an excellent time to do family therapy. For example, children, who may have reached adulthood can now express their feelings and experiences of living in an alcoholic family and in the early periods of recovery. For the first time, the family may be able to not only begin to process these distressing experiences and feelings, but to also experience reintegration into a new age-appropriate family system.

Some of the research families had adult children in the Ongoing Recovery Stage who were excited and proud of their recovering parents. They willingly engaged in family therapy and/or family meetings in order to strengthen healthy family attachments and family dynamics. In general, these children come from families in which both parents were in recovery and had significantly changed their addictive dynamics.

Other children went the route of acting out and/or using drugs or alcohol. These parents in recovery learned to not sacrifice their recovery for their children, but to establish clear boundaries, healthy communication, and emotional responsiveness toward them. Interestingly, some of these parents became role models for their chemically dependent children in this stage and supported them into sobriety.

CONCLUSION

Family recovery is still an unfamiliar concept in the field of addictions and alcoholism and as such, it has been the aim of this chapter to convey the "sense" of family recovery, to describe its profound complexities and difficulties, and to offer strategies to help negotiate through the stages of recovery. Family recovery is also a process with abstinence not marking the end, but the beginning of a journey that has no end–a realization that has caused alcoholics and co-alcoholics a certain degree of surprise and dismay (Brown & Lewis, 1999; Brown, Lewis, & Liotta, 2000). However, recovery is also a family promise to lifelong health with both change and growth being possible if both spouses accept responsibility for them (Lewis & Allen-Byrd, 2001).

Therapists who are knowledgeable about the dynamics of recovery from alcoholism can be very effective in forming appropriate treatment plans for families. Knowledge is power–the power to reduce relapses, to reduce confusion and pain, and to create timely assistance and coping strategies. This knowledge will help to normalize the recovery process and help families cope more successfully through bewildering times.

Therapists are also in a crucial position to help children who are typically relegated to the background by parents during the early recovery stage. Children are generally reluctant to voice their fears, resentments, confusion, because they feel guilty for having these feelings; particularly when they hear that recovery is so wonderful. They need as much attention and assistance as their parents if family recovery is to be fully successful. (Suggestions for working with children in each stage can be found in Brown, Lewis, & Liotta (2000).)

It is important for therapists and family members to understand that alcoholism is a family disease and that successful recovery is a family commitment which requires both spouses to be actively participating in treatment, self-responsibility, and adopting a long-term perspective on change in the self and the family (Lewis, Allen-Byrd, & Rouhbakhsh, 2004).

REFERENCES

Brown, S., Lewis, V., & Liotta, A. (2000). *The family recovery guide: A map for healthy growth.* Oakland, CA: New Harbinger Publications, Inc.

Brown, S., & Lewis, V. (1999). *The alcoholic family in recovery: A developmental model.* New York: Guilford Press.

Brown, S., & Lewis, V. (1995). The alcoholic family: A developmental model of recovery. In S. Brown & I. Yalom (Eds.). *Treating Alcoholism* (pp. 279-315). San Francisco: Jossey-Bass Publishers.

Lewis, V., Allen-Byrd, L., & Rouhbakhsh, P. (2004). Understanding successful family recovery: Two models. *Journal of Systemic Therapies, 23*(4), 39-51.

Lewis, V., & Allen-Byrd, L. (2001). The alcoholic family recovery typology. *Alcoholism Treatment Quarterly, 19*(3), 1-17.

doi:10.1300/J020v25n01_07

Treatment of Comorbidity in Families

Miriam Mulsow, PhD

SUMMARY. Half or more of all people presenting for treatment for alcohol disorders will also have an additional current or past psychological disorder. The presence of a comorbid disorder makes design and implementation of a treatment plan more complicated, completion of treatment less likely, and the odds of relapse greater. In addition, the presence of a comorbid disorder creates added stress on the social support network of the client, in particular, the client's family. In many cases, the stress reaches a level that leads to a cutoff between the client and family. However, when the family is still actively involved in the client's life, the family members may be able to provide much needed assistance in diagnosis, treatment, and support for abstinence. Current studies indicate that, in order to increase the likelihood of successful treatment, most comorbid disorders should be treated concurrently with alcohol disorders. doi:10.1300/J020v25n01_08 *[Article copies available for a fee from The Haworth Document Delivery Service: 1-800-HAWORTH. E-mail address: <docdelivery@haworthpress.com> Website: <http://www.HaworthPress.com> © 2007 by The Haworth Press, Inc. All rights reserved.]*

KEYWORDS. Alcohol, treatment, comorbidity, family, dual diagnosis

Miriam Mulsow is Associate Professor & Graduate Program Director, Dept. of Human Development and Family Studies, Texas Tech University, Box 41162, Lubbock, TX 79409-1162 (E-mail: miriam.mulsow@ttu.edu).

[Haworth co-indexing entry note]: "Treatment of Comorbidity in Families." Mulsow, Miriam. Co-published simultaneously in *Alcoholism Treatment Quarterly* (The Haworth Press, Inc.) Vol. 25, No. 1/2, 2007, pp. 125-140; and: *Familial Responses to Alcohol Problems* (ed: Judith L. Fischer, Miriam Mulsow, and Alan W. Korinek) The Haworth Press, Inc., 2007, pp. 125-140. Single or multiple copies of this article are available for a fee from The Haworth Document Delivery Service [1-800-HAWORTH, 9:00 a.m. - 5:00 p.m. (EST). E-mail address: docdelivery@haworthpress.com].

Available online at http://atq.haworthpress.com
© 2007 by The Haworth Press, Inc. All rights reserved.
doi:10.1300/J020v25n01_08

INTRODUCTION

For many families who have a member with alcohol disorders, difficulties are made even greater by the presence of one or more comorbid disorders. Community samples indicate that close to half of all people with alcohol disorders have comorbid disorders at the time of measurement (Helzer & Pryzbeck, 1988 in Ohannessian et al., 2004). This figure rises when examining the presence of a comorbid disorder at any time over the life course. In fact, Sonne and colleagues reported that 78.3% of men and 86% of women with a history of alcohol disorders met criteria for at least one other psychological disorder (Sonne, Back, Zuniga, Randall, & Brady, 2003).

According to West and colleagues, "clients in treatment for addictive disorders who present an additional psychiatric diagnosis are more likely to fail to engage in the treatment process, to leave treatment before completion, and to relapse after treatment" (West, Mulsow, & Arredondo, in press) than are patients without comorbid disorders. Thus, the family struggles with stressors associated with symptoms of two or more comorbid disorders, the demands of repeated attempts at treatment, plus the stigma attached to each (Daley & Marsill, 2005). Commonly, part of the stigma involves blame placed on the family for the presence of the disorders. It is not surprising, then, to learn that many families cut off contact with members who have alcohol disorders comorbid with other psychological disorders (MacDonald et al., 2004). However, when the family is available for participation in integrated family and alcohol or other drug use disorder treatment, improvements in both alcohol or other drug use and comorbid disorders are likely to be more lasting (Center for Substance Abuse Treatment, 2004).

Some comorbid disorders respond well to therapy or pharmacological treatment that is concurrent with treatment for addictions (Zimmerman, Sheeran, Chelminski, & Young, 2004). However, treatment for the comorbid disorder may need to continue after treatment for the alcohol disorder is completed (Wagner et al., 2004). There is sometimes a reluctance to use pharmacological intervention with clients who may be at risk to misuse medications. The present review will address disorders for which pharmacological intervention may be the most effective treatment as well as when this may not be needed. In addition, treatment professionals are faced with a dilemma when assessing and developing strategies for assisting clients with alcohol use disorders, because symptoms of alcohol use disorders and withdrawal can mimic those of psychological disorders (Samet, Nunes, & Hasin, 2004).

The family, if actively involved in the client's life, may be able to assist in diagnosis and treatment. For example, family members may be able to provide information concerning order of onset, so that the clinician will have a better idea of whether symptoms were caused by or existed prior to the alcohol or other drug disorder. In addition, the family may be able to assist the client in medication monitoring for the comorbid disorder (Center for Substance Abuse Treatment, 2004), or in parenting, when children are present or when the client is a minor (Center for Substance Abuse Treatment, 2005). When the identified patient is pregnant, the family may be enlisted to assist with medical needs prior to delivery and care for the newborn and mother after delivery. Commonly, pregnant women with comorbid alcohol and other disorders mistrust treatment professionals, perhaps fearing that they may lose custody of the baby after delivery (Center for Substance Abuse Treatment, 2005). Finally, the family may provide essential social support for abstinence, thus improving the client's chances for successfully moving into remission of the alcohol use and comorbid disorder (Evans & Sullivan, 1990, MacDonald et al., 2004).

The family needs to know that social support, which they may be in the best position to provide to the person in treatment, is the most important predictor of recovery from both alcohol and comorbid disorders (Evans & Sullivan, 1990; Fischer & Lyness, 2005; MacDonald et al., 2004). Social support also acts as a protective factor. People who are divorced, separated, or widowed experience a greater risk of comorbid alcohol and psychological disorders (Wang & El-Guebaly, 2004). Commonly, both the identified patient and the patient's family need to be taught how to have fun together (Evans & Sullivan, 1990).

Members of the family also need social support (Daley & Marsili, 2005). In addition to addiction-related sources of family support such as Al-Anon, families should be directed toward support groups for families of people with mental illness such as the National Alliance for the Mentally Ill (NAMI), when appropriate. These groups, as well as therapists working with the identified patient and family, should be able to help family members recognize the difference between appropriate support and enabling behaviors (Daley & Marsili, 2005).

When the family is engaged in the treatment process for comorbid alcohol and other disorders, one of the greatest needs that most families have is for information about both the alcohol disorder and the comorbid disorder as well as coping skills for dealing with these issues (Daley & Marsili, 2005). Families need to know that, without adequate treatment, one disorder can often exacerbate or "set off" the other (Center for

Substance Abuse Treatment, 2004). During the therapy process, families often need to address issues of anger, guilt, and grief over lost expectations and dreams. Unhealthy patterns of family interaction, as well as disorders occurring in other family members, may also require attention (Center for Substance Abuse Treatment, 2004). In addition, the family needs to be taught that recovery is a process, not an event, and that there may be lapses in recovery without complete relapse (Daley & Marsili, 2005; Evans & Sullivan, 1990). Thereby, the family will be better prepared to recognize, acknowledge, and encourage progress made even when lapses occur in alcohol disorders, in symptoms of comorbid disorders, or in both.

Among the more commonly encountered comorbid disorders with alcohol use disorders are Attention Deficit Hyperactivity Disorder, Post Traumatic Stress Disorder, subclinical symptoms associated with past abuse or other traumatic experiences, other Anxiety Disorders, and Mood Disorders. Each of these categories of disorders will be discussed in the present review. In addition, order of onset will be discussed as it influences treatment decisions (whether the alcohol use disorder or the comorbid disorder appeared first/was primary). Factors that may need to be considered in the development of treatment strategies for people with comorbid alcohol and other disorders include the client's cultural background, support system, and family history. Each of these factors will be briefly addressed.

There are other problems that are comorbid with alcohol use disorders and factors that influence treatment. No single review can cover all circumstances. However, information concerning the disorders and circumstances addressed in the present review may also be applicable when other situations arise.

COMORBID DISORDERS

Attention Deficit Hyperactivity Disorder

In a review of studies of Attention Deficit Hyperactivity Disorder (ADHD) and substance use disorders, Wilens states that ADHD is currently present in 25-31% of adolescents and 15-25% of adults presenting for alcohol or other drug disorder treatment (Wilens, 2004). Furthermore, ADHD is linked to earlier onset, longer recovery times, more severe alcohol or other drug disorder symptoms, and increased likelihood of failure in treatment (West et al., in press). A history of childhood ADHD was identified in 35-71% of adults with alcohol use disorders (Wilens, 2004). Presence or history of ADHD at least doubles the risk that a person will develop alcohol use disorders; 17-45% of adults with ADHD experience problems with alcohol use disorders (Wilens, 2004).

When one member of a family has ADHD, then there will usually be other biologically-related members of the family who have ADHD (Mulsow, O'Neal, & Murry, 2001). There is also a higher incidence of other psychological disorders among family members of people with ADHD (Wilens, 2004). The presence of several family members with ADHD and other disorders is likely to increase the number of stressors encountered by the family, reduce resources available to the family, and increase the likelihood that other members of the family will also be struggling with alcohol or other drug disorders (Mulsow et al., 2001; Wilens, 2004). Thus, for clients who live with such family members, environments may be chaotic and not conducive to recovery. Conversely, the client may have a family that is in a unique position to understand the struggles that he or she is facing and may, therefore, be an important source of social support through recovery.

Among adults with both ADHD and alcohol disorders, additional comorbid disorders are common (Wilens, 2004). Some studies suggest that the combination of ADHD and conduct or bipolar disorder may account for much of the association between ADHD and alcohol disorders. However, Wilens found that ADHD by itself also increased the risk of developing an alcohol or other drug use disorder.

When the ADHD is treated, outcome studies suggest that alcohol cravings may be reduced and treatment outcomes are somewhat improved (Wilens, 2004). The most effective treatment for ADHD involves the use of medication, and this concerns some practitioners. However, Wilens notes that "No evidence exists that treating ADHD pharmacologically through an active SUD [substance use disorder] exacerbates the SUD" (2004, p. 294). Treatment of alcohol and other drug disorders with comorbid ADHD is sometimes done concurrently; while in other cases, the alcohol or other drug disorder is addressed prior to directing attention toward the ADHD (Wilens, 2004). Symptoms of ADHD may lead to financial and employment problems, high levels of family stress, and weak or absent social support networks. Thus, the life of a client with severe, untreated ADHD may involve circumstances that lead to stigmatization and social isolation as well as association with groups that are more likely to support alcohol and other drug use than recovery. When ADHD is successfully treated, even with medication, many clients experience more success in recovering from alcohol and other drug disorders and in sustaining that recovery (Riggs, 1998; Schubiner et al., 1995).

It is important to note that the pharmacological treatment of ADHD in childhood reduces by about half the odds that the child will develop an alcohol or other drug use disorder in adolescence or adulthood (Wilens, 2004). Thus, the child becomes no more likely to develop such a disorder than a child without ADHD (Wilens, 2004). Because ADHD and alcohol use patterns are each commonly transmitted from one generation to the next, attention to ADHD symptoms among children of clients in treatment for alcohol disorders may be needed to provide protection against future alcohol or other drug use disorders in these children.

Post Traumatic Stress Disorder

Among those seeking treatment for alcohol or other drug use disorders, 38% of women and 17% of men met criteria for Post Traumatic Stress Disorder (PTSD), with rates even higher among adolescents (45.3% of females and 24.3% of males) (Sonne et al., 2003). Various types of trauma, among them a history of abuse or combat service, may cause PTSD. For example, a history of sexual abuse is more common among both males and females in treatment for alcohol and other drugs than in the general public (Lee, Mulsow, Fischer, Harris, Shumway, & Arredondo, 2004). The rate of sexual abuse history among women in treatment for alcohol and other drug disorders is particularly high (37.4% in the Lee et al., study).

Women with a history of sexual victimization tend to have lengthier and more repeated treatments, with clinicians reporting less cooperation in treatment among this group (Lee et al., 2004; Sonne et al., 2003). Alcohol or other drugs may be used as self-medication for the PTSD that results from sexual abuse. Alcohol use disorders prevent recovery from PTSD symptoms, thus providing a rationale for continued drinking (Stewart, Pihl, Conrod, & Dongier, 1998). In addition, Kilpatrick and colleagues describe a vicious cycle among women in which alcohol or other drug use increases the risk of future sexual assault and assault leads to an increase in alcohol or other drug use (Kilpatrick, Acierno, Resnick, Saunders, & Best, 1997). Furthermore, women with PTSD that is comorbid with alcohol or other drug use disorders are exposed to additional traumas related to the alcohol or other drug use disorder (Back, Sonne, Killeen, Dansky, & Brady, 2003).

Clinicians need to specifically ask women entering treatment for alcohol and other drug disorders about any history that they may have of sexual abuse (Lee et al., 2004), then address the sexual abuse concurrently with the alcohol or other drug disorder (Back et al., 2003). Root (1989) suggested that "the prevailing treatment goal of immediate abstinence from the problem substance before addressing the sexual assault and its aftermath is unrealistic and, indeed, destined for failure" (p. 543). Glover (1999) concurred, stating that when treatment for alcohol and other drug disorders does not address previous sexual victimization experiences, the potential for relapse increases. Because women's bodies are more seriously affected by alcohol disorders than are men's, including a greater likelihood of severe problems or death from alcohol-related causes (Back et al., 2003; Davis & DiNitto, 1996; Yaffe, Jenson, & Howard, 1995), attention to a history of sexual victimization is vital for women entering treatment.

People entering treatment for alcohol use disorders who have a history of physical or sexual abuse are also at risk for major depression that is then exacerbated by the pharmacological effects of alcohol on mood (Clark, De Bellis, Lynch, Cornelius, & Martin, 2003). Back and colleagues (2003) found that women who had comorbid PTSD and alcohol use disorders also had elevated rates of both depression and social phobia. Thus, when a history of abuse is identified, attention also should be given to the possibility of major depression and anxiety.

Women with a history of abuse are more likely to report that PTSD symptoms occurred before alcohol use disorders, whereas men report that alcohol use disorders occurred first (Sonne et al., 2003). Thus, women may be self-medicating the symptoms of PTSD, whereas men may be experiencing PTSD because of risky situations related to alcohol or other drug use. Among both men and women, avoidance of thoughts, feelings, and conversations about the trauma predicted worse treatment outcomes, suggesting that the trauma should be specifically addressed in treatment. Sonne and associates (2003) state that people with PTSD that predates alcohol use disorders should be treated first for the trauma, whereas people with alcohol use disorders that predate PTSD should be treated first for the addiction. As these are commonly gender related, Sonne and associates suggest that specific intake procedures be developed for males and females with alcohol use disorders.

Although PTSD is more common among women than men in treatment for alcohol disorders (Center for Substance Abuse Treatment, 2005), both women and men with PTSD are at greater risk for alcohol disorders.

When men present with comorbid PTSD and alcohol disorders, the source of the PTSD is most commonly combat or politically-related violence (Center for Substance Abuse Treatment, 2005). Clients with combat-related PTSD are likely to be more verbally and physically aggressive than other clients (Zoricic, Karlovic, Buljan, & Marusic, 2003). This aggression commonly leads to marital difficulties as well as antisocial behaviors, both of which lead to a loss of family support for the client as well as an increase in stress for the family. Many veteran's hospitals have PTSD treatment units that address both the trauma and the subsequent substance abuse (Center for Substance Abuse Treatment, 2005).

Other Anxiety Disorders

It has been suggested that clinicians recognize and intervene more effectively in cases of depression comorbid with alcohol disorders than in cases of anxiety comorbid with alcohol disorders (Haver, 2003). However, anxiety and alcohol use disorders are commonly comorbid (Marquez, Seugi, Cane, Garcia, & Ortiz, 2003). In fact, alcohol may have a "kindling effect" on the emergence of panic disorder (Marquez et al., 2003). Schuckit and colleagues found a three-fold or higher risk for panic disorder and social phobia among people with alcohol use disorders (Schuckit et al., 1997). Both males and females in treatment for alcohol use disorders report social anxiety disorders and state that they drink in order to relieve social and performance anxiety (Randall, Thomas, & Thevos, 2000). When women in treatment for alcohol use disorders have comorbid phobic disorders, they are more likely to drop out of treatment and, therefore, have poorer outcomes in both drinking and mental health (Haver, 2003). If screening for social anxiety disorders is a routine part of every intake, and treatment for social anxiety is concurrent with treatment for the alcohol use disorder, then social anxiety disorders can be recognized and treatments can be tailored to the needs of these clients, thus increasing the chances for sustained recovery (Randall et al., 2000). In addition, Randall and colleagues indicate that both males and females with comorbid anxiety and alcohol use disorders report family and social problems. They suggest that people with comorbid social anxiety and alcohol disorders may benefit from family therapy that teaches skills in communication and social interactions.

Mood Disorders

Alcohol and drug use disorders and major depression tend to co-occur (Grant & Dawson, 1999). As with a history of trauma, social anxiety, and ADHD, concurrent treatment for mood disorders may improve alcohol disorder treatment outcome. Unlike ADHD, Hesse reports that medication may not be needed for reducing alcohol or other drug disorders in clients with comorbid depression if Cognitive Behavioral Therapy (CBT) is available and the patient responds to this treatment (Hesse, 2004). When there is a strong positive relationship between the client and family, involvement of the family in some stages of therapy may improve the chances of successfully treating mood disorders. Either medication or CBT helped to reduce alcohol or other drug use in clients with comorbid depression, but combining the two treatments did not improve outcomes (Hesse, 2004).

Major depression could occur either before or after the onset of alcohol use disorders for women, but tended to occur after the onset of alcohol use disorders for men (de Graaf, Bijl, Spijker, Beekman, & Vollegergh, 2003). Dysthymia tended to occur before the onset of alcohol use disorders for women but was somewhat more likely to occur after the onset of alcohol use disorders for men. Bipolar disorder tended to occur after the onset of alcohol use disorders in women but was somewhat more likely to occur before the onset of alcohol use disorders for men (de Graaf, et al., 2003). Men with mood disorders appear to be at a particularly elevated risk for alcohol or other drug disorders. For example, de Graaf and colleagues (2003) report that 56.5% of men with bipolar disorder, 40.6% of men with dysthymia, and 43.1% of men with major depression had some form of alcohol or other drug disorder diagnosed over the course of their lives. However, only 29.7% of women with bipolar disorder, 16.1% of women with dysthymia, and 14.4% of women with major depression had some form of alcohol or other drug use disorder diagnosed at some time in their lives (de Graaf et al., 2003). Conversely, de Graaf and associates report that when women had alcohol use disorders, they were much more likely to also have some form of lifetime mood disorder than were men.

In young males, this link between mood and alcohol use disorders was not significant (de Graaf et al., 2003), possibly because heavy use of alcohol is more accepted for this group. Mood disorders were more commonly comorbid with anxiety disorders than with alcohol or other drug use disorders in both genders. Anxiety tended to precede mood disorders, but mood disorders could either precede or follow alcohol or other drug use disorders (de Graaf et al., 2003).

Because mood disorders contribute to relationship problems, and social support is important in treatment for alcohol disorders, when a client presents with comorbid mood and alcohol disorders, the mood disorder should be given attention in treatment. Treatment for the mood disorders may help in the process of healing family relationships, which may, in turn, help the client to recover from the alcohol disorder. When the mood disorder occurs before the alcohol disorder, then alcohol may be a form of self-medication. Thus, successful treatment for the mood disorder may reduce the client's perceived need for alcohol in addition to improving family relationships. Treatment for the mood disorder may make treatment for the alcohol disorder more effective. Order of onset and its implications will be discussed in the following section.

ISSUES THAT MAY INFLUENCE COMORBID DISORDERS OR THEIR TREATMENT

Order of Onset: Primary versus Secondary Disorders

In discussions of comorbid alcohol and other disorders, there is emphasis on the importance of primary and secondary disorders. The distinction between the two is based on both age of onset (which came first) and whether the disorders are thought to be independent or related. A disorder does not have to be caused by the primary disorder to be considered secondary, according to Samet et al. (2004). A disorder can be "chronologically secondary, regardless of the nature of the relationships between the primary and secondary disorders (Samet et al., 2004, p. 10)."

However, when addressing a primary disorder with secondary alcohol disorder, the terminology is usually applied to mean that the symptoms of the primary disorder are not caused by the alcohol or its effects. A primary disorder must be ruled out before a substance-induced disorder can be diagnosed. According to Samet and colleagues (2004), a primary disorder must meet one of these criteria: (a) has symptoms well beyond what would be expected to be linked to the alcohol or other drug or withdrawal from the alcohol or other drug, (b) history of symptoms of the disorder that are not linked to the alcohol or other drug, (c) onset before onset of alcohol or other drug use disorder, or (d) symptoms remain at least a month after intoxication and withdrawal have completely ceased. When none of these criteria are met, then the symptoms are assumed to be related to the alcohol or other drug use or withdrawal. This replaces the chronologically primary versus secondary criteria, because the disorder may have existed but not been diagnosed prior to the client entering treatment for the alcohol disorder (Samet et al., 2004). However, Samet and colleagues find that the criteria: "has symptoms well beyond what would be expected to be linked to the substance or withdrawal from the substance," is problematic in that "beyond what would be expected" is not defined. In the ICD-10, the international version of DSM-IV, there is no such issue. A disorder is either "organic" or substance induced and cannot be both.

The family may be particularly helpful in determining whether symptoms of a comorbid disorder are caused by the alcohol disorder or are independent of that disorder. They may be able to tell the clinician when symptoms first appeared and whether symptoms of the comorbid disorder(s) remained during extended periods of abstinence (Center for Substance Abuse Treatment, 2005). In addition, a family medical history may tell the clinician whether the comorbid disorder is present in other family members who do not have alcohol use disorders.

Culture and Ethnicity Background

Culture, ethnicity, and context each influence the occurrence of alcohol use and comorbid disorders. For example, in the US, ethnicity strongly predicts alcohol use disorders, with the highest usage found among white males. In Spain, a country in which alcohol use begins at an early age, alcohol disorders tend to preceed comorbid disorders (Marquez et al., 2003). In the Netherlands, alcohol use disorders tend to arise in the mid-twenties for males and the later twenties for females (de Graaf et al., 2003). Determining which disorder is primary and which is secondary may be easier in cultures in which alcohol use tends to begin later. However, "comorbidities between psychiatric and substance-use disorders are relevant across countries and cultures" (Samet et al., 2004, p. 9).

Unlike the general population of the United States, men of Mexican origin, as a group, do not experience the decline in heavy drinking that occurs after age 29 (Vega, Sribney, & Achara-Abrahams, 2003). Thus, men of Mexican origin experience higher rates of alcohol related diseases and deaths. The problems are worse among more acculturated men than among more recent immigrants. The same situation exists for women of Mexican origin, with those born in the United States being five times more likely to experience alcohol use disorders than those born in Mexico. However, alcohol disorder rates for women of both groups are low. Immigrant men of Mexican origin who had comorbid disorders were likely to have alcohol plus another drug use disorder. US born men and women of Mexican origin who had comorbid disorders were likely to have a nonsubstance disorder in addition to alcohol and other drug disorders. Immigrant women of Mexican origin had negligible alcohol or other drug use disorders. (Vega et al., 2003).

It may be useful to ask clients of Mexican origin where they were born. Sensitivity should be shown, however, for any concerns clients may have about immigration status. For clients who are second or subsequent generation, followup treatment for the alcohol disorder may need to continue for longer periods than that for more recent immigrants. Given the importance of extended family as a primary source of support for persons of Mexican origin, members of the extended family should be asked to participate in treatment whenever possible, with attention given to members of the extended family who may also struggle with alcohol and other disorders.

Support System

The presence of a strong social support network provides a protective factor for people with psychological disorders or alcohol disorders. When abstinence occurs, strengthening of social support for abstinence tends to precede reduction in consumption (MacDonald et al., 2004). Similarly, a descent into alcohol and other drug misuse tends to be associated with a reduction in social support from family and an increase in support from peers who encourage use. MacDonald and associates suggest that people with psychological disorders may use substances as a way to help them increase their social support networks. Therefore, they fear recovery because of the potential loss of social support from substance-using peers. However, as their disorders progress, they tend to lose even the substance using peer network (MacDonald et al., 2004). As people with comorbid disorders progress through stages of treatment, they perceive more support from professionals and seem to value this support more (MacDonald et al., 2004).

Family History

Family history influences the presence or absence of comorbid disorders. For example, Ohannessian and associates (2004) found that adolescents whose parents had alcohol use disorders only were no more likely to have psychological disorders than were adolescents whose parents had no known disorders. However, if the parents had comorbid drug dependence or depression, then the adolescents were more likely to have psychological disorders. If the parents had both drug dependence and depression, then the adolescents were the most likely to have psychological disorders. Specifically, children of parents with comorbid alcohol use disorders and a psychological disorder were at increased risk for conduct disorder, depression, and alcohol and other drug use disorders compared to adolescents whose parents had no lifetime psychopathology. The effects of paternal disorders appeared to be stronger than the effects of maternal disorders, but this might have been due to low statistical power in the group of mothers. There might not have been enough mothers in the sample to detect significant relationships between the variables for mothers (Ohannessian et al., 2004).

Children of alcohol dependent parents do not have an elevated risk for conduct disorder, depression, or early onset alcohol or marijuana dependence unless their parents have a history of comorbid disorders (Ohannessian et al., 2004). "Multiple risk factors increase an individual's probability of developing psychological problems" (Ohannessian et al., p. 529). The authors suggest that the reason for this may be genetic, environmental, or a combination of both. In terms of environmental explanations, parents with comorbid alcohol use disorders and other psychological disorders may have more family and employment problems, leading to a more stressful environment for their children. Alternatively, family and employment problems and associated family stress may contribute to both comorbid disorders in the parents and elevated risk for the children (Ohannessian et al., 2004). In the Ohannessian et al., study, 67% of fathers and 75% of mothers with alcohol use disorders had comorbid depression, drug dependence, or both. Only 20% of fathers and 9% of mothers had alcohol use disorders only. If their sample is typical of parents with alcohol disorders, then a high proportion of families affected by alcohol disorders also face stressors associated with comorbid disorders.

CONCLUSIONS

Although rates varied across studies, all of the studies that examined comorbid disorders among people with alcohol disorders found a high incidence of comorbid disorders, and many researchers found these in a majority of participants. For most disorders, concurrent treatment for alcohol disorders and comorbid disorders was recommended. Haver suggested that, "optimal treatment of psychiatric disorders among subjects with drinking problems" (2003, p. 42) is important to both quality of life and recurrence of drinking. Because many persons with comorbid alcohol and other disorders live with families members that also have these conditions, clinicians should consider attending to the needs of family members and exploring the potential support for abstinence that these family members may be able to offer. Furthermore, attention to children of parents with alcohol and comorbid disorders may help to prevent the intergenerational transmission of some of these disorders.

REFERENCES

Back, S. E., Sonne, S. C., Killeen, T., Dansky, B. S., & Brady, K. T. (2003). Comparative profiles of women with PTSD and comorbid cocaine or alcohol dependence. *The American Journal of Drug and Alcohol Abuse, 29,* 169-189.

Center for Substance Abuse Treatment (2004). *Substance abuse treatment and family therapy.* Treatment Improvement Protocol (TIP) Series, No. 39. DHHS Publication No. (SMA) 04 -3957. Rockville, MD: Substance Abuse and Mental Health Services Administration.

Center for Substance Abuse Treatment (2005). *Substance abuse treatment for persons with co-occurring disorders.* Treatment Improvement Protocol (TIP) Series, No. 42. DHHS Publication No. (SMA) 05-3922. Rockville, MD: Substance Abuse and Mental Health Services Administration.

Clark, D. B., De Bellis, M. D., Lynch, K. G., Cornelius, J. R., & Martin, C. S. (2003). Physical and sexual abuse, depression and alcohol use disorders in adolescents: Onsets and outcomes. *Drug and Alcohol Dependence, 69,* 51-60.

Daley, D. C., & Marsili, R. (2005). No one is left unharmed: Dual disorders and the family. *Counselor, 6,* 37-44.

Davis, D. R., & DiNitto, D. M. (1996). Gender differences in social and psychological problems of substance abusers: A comparison to nonsubstance abusers. *Journal of Psychoactive Drugs, 28,* 135-145.

de Graaf, R., Bijl, R. V., Spijker, J., Beekman, A. T. F., & Vollegergh, W. A. M. (2003). Temporal sequencing of lifetime mood disorders in relation to comorbid anxiety and substance use disorders: Findings from the Netherlands Mental Health Survey and Incidence Study. *Social Psychiatry and Psychiatric Epidemiology, 38,* 1-11.

Evans, K., & Sullivan, J. M. (1990). *Dual diagnosis: Counseling the mentally ill substance abuser.* New York: Guilford Press.

Fischer, J., & Lyness, K. P. (2005). Families coping with alcohol and substance abuse. in P. C. McKenry & S. J. Price (Eds) *Families and change: Coping with stressful events and transitions (3rd Ed),* pp. 155-178. Thousand Oaks, CA: Sage Publications.

Glover, N. M. (1999). Play therapy and art therapy for substance abuse clients who have a history of incest victimization. *Journal of Substance Abuse Treatment, 16,* 281-287.

Grant, B. F. & Dawson, D. A. (1999). Alcohol and drug use, abuse, and dependence: Classification, prevalence, and comorbidity. In B.S. McGrady & E. E. Epstein, (Eds.), *Addictions: A comprehensive guidebook* (pp. 9-29). NY: Oxford University Press.

Haver, B. (2003). Comorbid psychiatric disorders predict and influence treatment outcome in female alcoholics. *European Addiction Research, 9,* 39-44.

Hesse, M. (2004). Achieving abstinence by treating depression in the presence of substance-use disorders. *Addictive Behaviors, 29,* 1137-1141.

Kilpatrick, D. G., Acierno, R., Resnick, H. S., Saunders, B. E., & Best, C. L. (1997). A 2-year longitudinal analysis of the relationships between violent assault and substance use in women. *Journal of Consulting and Clinical Psychology, 65,* 834-847.

Lee, J. R., Mulsow, M., Fischer, J., Harris, K., Shumway, S., & Arredondo, R. (2004). Effects of gender, sexual victimization, and duration of alcohol and other drug abuse on treatment history. *Alcoholism Treatment Quarterly, 22,* 27-42.

Marquez, M., Seugi, J., Cane, J., Garcia, L., & Ortiz, M. (2003). Alcoholism in 274 patients with panic disorder in Spain, One of the main producers of wine worldwide. *Journal of Affective Disorders, 75,* 237-246.

MacDonald, E. M., Luxmore, M., Pica, S., Tanti, C., Blackman, J. M., Catford, N., & Stockton, P. (2004). Social networks of people with dual diagnosis: The quantity and quality of relationships at different stages of substance use treatment. *Community Mental Health Journal, 40,* 451-464.

Mulsow, M., O'Neal, K. K., & Murry, V. M. (2001) Adult Attention Deficit Hyperactivity Disorder, the family, and child maltreatment. *Trauma, Violence, & Abuse, 2,* 36-50.

Ohannessian, C. M., Hesselbrock, V. M., Kramer, J., Kuperman, S., Bucholz, K. K., Schuckit, M. A., & Nurnberger, J. I. (2004). The relationship between parental alcoholism and adolescent psychopathology: A systematic examination of parental comorbid psychopathology. *Journal of Abnormal Child Psychology, 32,* 519-533.

Randall, C. L., Thomas, S. E., & Thevos, A. K. (2000). Gender comparison in alcoholics with concurrent social phobia: Implications for alcoholism treatment. *The American Journal on Addictions, 9,* 202-215.

Riggs, P. D. (1998). Clinical approach to treatment of ADHD in adolescents with substance use disorders and conduct disorders. *Journal of the American Academy of Child and Adolescent Psychiatry, 37,* 331-332.

Root, M. P. (1989). Treatment failures: The role of sexual victimization in women's addictive behavior. *American Journal of Orthopsychiatry, 59,* 542-548.

Samet, S., Nunes, E. V., & Hasin, D. (2004). Diagnosing comorbidity: Concepts, criteria, and methods. *Acta Neuropsychitrica, 16,* 9-18.

Schubiner, H., Tzelepis, A., Isaacson, J. H., Warbasse, L. H., Zacharek, M., & Musial, J. (1995). The dual diagnosis of attention-deficit/hyperactivity disorder and substance abuse: Case reports and literature review. *Journal of Clinical Psychiatry, 56,* 146-150.

Schuckit, M. A., Tipp, J. E., Bucholz, K. K., Nurnberger, J. I. Jr, Hesselbrock, V. M, Crowe, R. R., et al. (1997). The life-time rates of three major mood disorders and four major anxiety disorders in alcoholics and controls, *Addiction, 92,* 1289-1304.

Sonne, S. C., Back, S. E., Zuniga, C. D., Randall, C. L., & Brady, K. T. (2003). Gender differences in individuals with comorbid alcohol dependence and post-traumatic stress disorder. *The American Journal on Addictions, 12*, 412-423.

Stewart, S. H., Pihl, R. O., Conrod, P. J., & Dongier, M. (1998). Functional associations among trauma, PTSD, and substance-related disorders. *Addictive Behavior, 23*, 797-812.

Vega, W. A., Sribney, M. S., & Achara-Abrahams, I. (2003). Co-occurring alcohol, drug, and other psychiatric disorders among Mexican-origin people in the United States. *American Journal of Public Health, 93*, 1057-1064.

Wagner, T., Krampe, H., Stawicki, S., Reinhold, J., Jahn, H., Mahlke, K., et al. (2004). Substantial decrease of psychiatric comorbidity in chronic alcoholics upon integrated outpatient treatment-Results of a prospective study. *Journal of Psychiatric Research, 38*, 619-635.

Wang, J. L., & El-Guebaly, N. (2004). Sociodemographic factors associated with comorbid major depressive episodes and alcohol dependence in the general population. *Canadian Journal of Psychiatry, 49*, 37-44.

West, S., Mulsow, M., & Arredondo, R. (in press). An examination of the psychometric properties of the Attention Deficit Scales for Adults with outpatient substance abusers. *American Journal of Drug and Alcohol Abuse, 31*.

Wilens, T. E. (2004). Attention-deficit hyperactivity disorder and the substance use disorders: The nature of the relationship, subtypes at risk, and treatment issues. *Psychiatric Clinics of North America, 27*, 283-301.

Yaffe, J. Jenson, J. M. & Howard, M. O. (1995). Women and substance abuse: Implications for treatment. *Alcoholism Treatment Quarterly, 13*, 1-15.

Zimmerman, M., Sheeran, T., Chelminski, I., & Young, D. (2004). Screening for psychiatric disorders in outpatients with DSM-IV substance use disorders. *Journal of Substance Abuse Treatment, 26*, 181-188.

Zoricic, Z., Korlovic, D., Buljan, D., & Marusic, S. (2003). Comorbid alcohol addiction increases aggression level in soldiers with combat-related post-traumatic stress disorder. *Nordic Journal of Psychiatry, 57*, 199-202.

doi:10.1300/J020v25n01_08

Promoting Spirituality in Families
with Alcoholism

Alan W. Korinek, PhD

SUMMARY. The role of spirituality in the etiology, progression, and treatment of alcoholism has been discussed and explored for some time now. In most of those discussions, it is the spirituality of the individual that has been the focus. This paper presents the concept of a "family spirituality" and discusses the effects of alcoholism on that spirituality. Suggestions are given regarding spiritually-based practices that clinicians can employ to heal and enhance the spirituality of the family that has been affected by alcohol. A case example is included. doi:10.1300/J020v25n01_09 *[Article copies available for a fee from The Haworth Document Delivery Service: 1-800-HAWORTH. E-mail address: <docdelivery@haworthpress.com> Website: <http://www.HaworthPress.com> © 2007 by The Haworth Press, Inc. All rights reserved.]*

KEYWORDS. Alcoholism, spirituality, substance abuse treatment, spiritual practices

---

Alan W. Korinek is Director of the Employee Assistance Program, Southwest Institute for Addictive Diseases, Texas Tech University Health Sciences Center, Lubbock, TX.

Address correspondence to: Alan W. Korinek, PhD, Texas Tech University Health Sciences Center, Department of Neuropsychiatry, 3601 4th Street, STOP 8103, Lubbock, TX 79430 (E-mail: alan.korinek@ttuhsc.edu).

[Haworth co-indexing entry note]: "Promoting Spirituality in Families with Alcoholism." Korinek, Alan W. Co-published simultaneously in *Alcoholism Treatment Quarterly* (The Haworth Press, Inc.) Vol. 25, No. 1/2, 2007, pp. 141-157; and: *Familial Responses to Alcohol Problems* (ed: Judith L. Fischer, Miriam Mulsow, and Alan W. Korinek) The Haworth Press, Inc., 2007, pp. 141-157. Single or multiple copies of this article are available for a fee from The Haworth Document Delivery Service [1-800-HAWORTH, 9:00 a.m. - 5:00 p.m. (EST). E-mail address: docdelivery@haworthpress.com].

Available online at http://atq.haworthpress.com
© 2007 by The Haworth Press, Inc. All rights reserved.
doi:10.1300/J020v25n01_09

INTRODUCTION

Alcohol abuse and addiction are multifaceted, multidimensional problems, with profound biological and sociological roots. In the opinion of many scholars and authors (e.g., Gorsuch, 1993; Kurtz, 1979; Miller, 1990), spirituality also plays a role in the etiology and progression of alcoholism. Spirituality provides a vital resource for healing and recovery. There is a growing body of literature supporting the notion that healthy spirituality is an important component in reducing the incidence of disease and in coping successfully with various kinds of problems, including alcoholism (Larson, Swyers, & McCullough, 1997; Martin & Carlson, 1988).

In this article, spiritual issues in the family of the alcoholic will be addressed. The concept of a "family spirituality" will be discussed, as well as the effects of alcoholism on that spirituality. Several spiritual practices will be presented that have the potential to heal and enhance the spirituality of families affected by alcoholism.

DEFINING SPIRITUALITY

Despite the evidence supporting the inclusion of spirituality as a component in treatment, change has been slow. There are historic barriers, including the separation of the sacred from the secular and the schism between faith-based and scientific approaches to health and healing. Another possible barrier is the lack of consensus regarding how spirituality should be defined.

A myriad of definitions of spirituality have been set forth by proponents. When examined, however, several themes usually emerge. One theme is that spirituality involves connectedness. For example, Perry and Rolland (1999) asserted that "Spirituality...involves the awareness that at the heart of things, at the heart of human existence and of all creation, there is a profound interconnectedness, an intricate interdependence" (p. 274). A second theme common to many definitions is that spirituality involves making meaning and/or searching for meaning (Kurtz & Ketcham, 1992). A third theme, absent in some definitions of spirituality, but prominent in others, is the presence of a transcendent being or higher power. This transcendent being or higher power is believed to play a role in the creation of connection and the discovery of meaning. Thus, Anderson (1999) defined spirituality as "the experience of making meaning informed by a relationship with the transcendent or divine in life" (p. 157). Fukuyama and Sevig (1997) agreed that a search for meaning and a relationship with the divine both could be part of a person's spirituality.

Although the inability to clearly define and operationalize spirituality may increase skepticism in some, others see that reality as reassuring. Kurtz and Ketcham (1992) stated, "When we attempt to 'define' spirituality, we discover not its limits, but our own...Timeless wisdom suggests that spirituality can't be proven; it can't be defined; it is elusive, ineffable, unbounded" (p. 16). Other authors (e.g., Miller, 1999) also contend that spirituality is multidimensional and complex, making it difficult to define.

Although many authors see an association between spirituality and the divine, there is much debate about the relationship between spirituality and another concept commonly associated with the divine, namely religion. In the opinion of many authors (e.g., Kurtz & Ketcham, 1992; Miller & Thoresen, 1999; Walsh, 1999), spirituality and religion are related, yet separate concepts, and it is important to differentiate between them. Other authors (e.g., Carlson & Erickson, 2000) are reluctant to make too clear a distinction between spirituality and religion. In Brawer et al.'s (2002) study, they combined the two words as religion/spirituality to provide participants with the broadest possible interpretation.

Where most advocates of spirituality appear to be in agreement is around the issue of the universality of spirituality. Human beings, in addition to being biological, psychological, and social creatures, are spiritual by nature, and spirituality is a part of each person (Aponte, 1999; Kurtz & Ketcham, 1992; Miller, 1999; Miller & Thoresen, 1999). "Spirituality is a lot like health...We may have good health or poor health, but it's something we can't avoid having...The question is...whether the spirituality we have is a negative one that leads to isolation and self-destruction or one that is more positive and life-giving" (Jerome Dollard, quoted in Kurtz & Ketcham, 1992, p. 17).

ALCOHOLISM AND SPIRITUALITY

Carl Jung was one of the first to propose a spiritual explanation for the development of alcoholism, suggesting that alcoholics were individuals who had a greater thirst for the spirit than others (Peck, 1993). Similar explanations offered more recently are that alcoholics, through their use of alcohol, are attempting to fulfill their longing for God (May, 1988), find their way into Paradise (Peck, 1993), or meet general spiritual needs that cannot be met through a materialistic culture (Royce, 1995). Evidence supporting the hypothesis that alcoholism is a spiritual condition is provided by the success of Alcoholics Anonymous (AA), a spiritual program that introduces its adherents to the concept of a higher power. From its beginnings, AA experienced much greater success in treating alcoholism than the traditional approaches were achieving (Peck, 1993). The "Big Book" of AA asserts that alcoholism is "an illness which only a spiritual experience will conquer" (*Alcoholics Anonymous*, 1976, p. 44). Through his psychiatric treatment of addicts, Peck (1993) discovered that greater success could be achieved by emphasizing the progressive aspects of the disorder, namely, the yearning for the spirit and for God.

Despite the success of spiritual approaches like AA, many researchers and clinicians continued to overlook the role that spiritual beliefs and practices might play in discouraging substance abuse and relapse (Gorsuch, 1995). However, when the available research on the relationship of spirituality to alcohol and drug problems was reviewed by a panel convened in conjunction with the National Institute for Healthcare Research, the panel concluded that there is strong evidence that spiritual involvement predicts less use of and fewer problems with alcohol, tobacco, and illicit drugs (Larson et al., 1997).

SPIRITUALITY AS A RELATIONAL CONSTRUCT

Spirituality is viewed primarily as something belonging to and experienced by the individual. However, spirituality can also be conceptualized as a relational construct (Anderson, 1999). Although it is an attribute of individuals, spirituality is also a component of relationships so that we can speak of "interpersonal spirituality" as well as "intrapersonal spirituality." Anderson (1999) stated, "Soul...is simultaneously individual and communal" (p. 160).

The family is an important communal relationship. Anderson (1999) asserted that families possess a communal soul. Regarding that communal soul, he stated, "Soul is what gives a living organism like a family unity and direction, making the parts into a composite whole, uniting with others and with the divine" (Anderson, 1999, p. 160). Thus, we can speak of both spirituality in the family and "family spirituality." The first concerns the spirituality of individual family members and might be assessed by using individual measures of spirituality. Family spirituality, on the other hand, has to do with the spirituality evidenced in the relationships within the family.

Although family spirituality is related to the spirituality of the individuals in the family, it is more than just the sum of the individuals' spiritualities. Thus if one partner in a couple has a spirituality that is healthy and the spirituality of the other person is unhealthy, the relationship will not be "half spiritual." Indeed, the degree of difference between them may create significant conflict, resulting in a relationship that is spiritually unhealthy and a communal soul that is damaged or perhaps "lost." Healthy individual spirituality promotes an awareness of interpersonal spirituality and a desire to improve it (Perry & Rolland, 1999).

EFFECTS OF ALCOHOLISM ON FAMILY SPIRITUALITY

There are many threats to family spirituality. Cultural values that function as "competing spiritualities" include individualism, consumerism, violence, professionalism, and despair (Perry & Rolland, 1999, p. 289). Overindulgence, a by-product of consumerism, also poses a serious threat, particularly when it leads to addictions (Martin & Booth, 1999).

Alcoholism, in particular, can have a profound effect on family spirituality (May, 1991). As the disease of alcoholism progresses, the alcoholic develops an intolerance of others, characterized by suspicion, distrust, and frequent arguments, as well as feelings of estrangement, alienation, and loneliness (Royce, 1995). Finnegan and McNally (1995) stated, "The downward descent into alcoholism is a descent into a hell of loss–loss of faith in a God who cares; loss of connection with any God or power outside of self; loss of connection with others and with self" (p. 42).

Steinglass, Bennett, Wolin, and Reiss (1987) wrote about "the Alcoholic Family," which they defined as a family where "behaviors related to alcohol use have come to play a major role within both morphogenetic and morphostatic mechanisms of the family system" (p. 46). The authors contended that in families where that situation exists, it is possible to say that the entire family has alcoholism. Alcohol invades the family and insidiously attacks its spiritual foundation, severely damaging the communal soul. Because the process is gradual, with accommodations to alcoholism made one small increment at a time, it is often the case that the amount of spiritual damage inflicted upon the family is not apparent until later. Indicators of spiritual damage include an overwhelming sense of ennui and emotional distance (Steinglass et al., 1987) and the creation of destructive entitlement, evidenced by double binds, family secrets, domination, and cutoffs, all of which deplete the trust resources in the family (Hargrave, 1994).

Alcoholism affects three areas of family life in particular: daily routines, family rituals, and short-term problem-solving strategies (Steinglass et al., 1987). Alcoholism's impact on family rituals, particularly family celebrations (e.g., weddings, funerals, religious holidays) and family traditions (e.g., summer vacations, birthday and anniversary customs) seems to be the most indicative of the attack on the family's spirituality. "By admitting alcohol into this inner sanctum of family life, the family allows its identity to change" (Steinglass et al., 1987, p. 233). Since a family's values are often conserved and reinforced through its rituals (Imber-Black & Roberts, 1992), allowing alcoholism to invade this important area sends a powerful message about the centrality of the disease.

PROMOTING HEALTHY FAMILY SPIRITUALITY

Addressing spirituality issues and encouraging spiritual growth in the family can provide great benefits for family health. Family process research has found that transcendent spiritual beliefs and practices are key ingredients in healthy family functioning (Beavers & Hampson, 1990; Stinnett & DeFrain, 1985). In a qualitative study conducted with families of children with disabilities, participants spoke very passionately about their spiritual beliefs as a contributor to their emotional and overall family quality of life (Poston & Turnbull, 2004). Similarly, addressing spirituality issues in the family provides hope for restoring a communal soul damaged by alcoholism (May, 1991).

A growing body of research underscores the efficacy of involving families in the treatment of alcoholism (Samford et al., 2001; Steinglass, Tislenko, & Reiss, 1985). Edwards and Steinglass (1995) stated, "An unbiased reading of [the research literature on family factors and alcoholism] suggests that active involvement of families, especially spouses, as an important component of a comprehensive treatment approach would be a reasonable and prudent direction to take" (p. 475). Although the communal soul of the family may be enhanced as a result of the alcoholic addressing his or her spirituality issues individually, involving the family in interventions designed to affect the family's spirituality increases the probability that the communal soul will be touched and transformed.

Many spiritually-based practices and exercises commonly used with individuals can be employed also by families, and several will be presented now. Prior to recommending these exercises to clients, however, clinicians should examine their own beliefs and biases regarding spirituality. At a minimum, the clinician must be open to the possibility that the family will be helped by being invited and encouraged to address spirituality issues. Ideally, clinicians are engaged in their own program of spiritual growth. Professionals who commit themselves to spiritual health and growth are in a much better position to help families whose members are attempting to address issues regarding their spirituality.

Clinicians eager to address spirituality issues with families should keep in mind a few cautions. In most cases, clinicians must operate with a definition of spirituality that is broad, inclusive and diverse (Finnegan & McNally, 1995), being careful not to promote specific belief systems (Poston & Turnbull, 2004). At the same time, clinicians must be prepared for clients' anger at God, their cynicism, and even their rejection of God, since many of these feelings are common in the face of trauma (Finnegan & McNally, 1995).

The clinician must always consider where the family is with regard to their comfort level with spirituality issues. Some of the spiritual activities promoted here may be engaged in more easily, especially for families who have neglected their spirituality or have been opposed to "spiritual" activities or practices. A kind of readiness is required before some spiritual activities can be entered into meaningfully, and if it is lacking, the engagement could do more harm than good, particularly if the family is pressured into being spiritual. Families must be encouraged to devote time and energy to the development of spiritual disciplines and practices. If they have not been accustomed to engaging in activities related to spiritual growth, they will need to be patient with one another and the clinician will need to be patient with them.

Meditation

The first spirituality-enhancing behavior to be discussed is meditation. Although often thought of as an individual activity, families also can engage in corporate meditation that heals and strengthens the communal soul. "Shared meditative experiences foster authentic and empathic communication, reduce defensive reactivity, and can deepen couple and family bonds" (Walsh, 1999, p. 44).

One of the great benefits of meditation seems to be its invitation to be still and listen. Anderson (1999) declared, "The way of the soul is passivity. We are human when we wait as well as when we act" (p. 159). There is a great temptation to "be busy" at all times and when one succumbs to that temptation, there is little time for reflection. One of the possible reasons alcoholics are determined to stay busy is that it distracts them from the negative, shaming self-talk that can fill times of stillness. Meditation and reflection require listening, especially listening to the spirit within and the Spirit that is one's higher power.

Kus (1995) described two types of meditation. The first, meditation as reflection, is very common in 12-step programs. It typically entails the use of meditation books that invite the reader to reflect on a particular concept or virtue or defect and how it applies to her or his life. Many of these books have meditations for each day of the year. The second type of meditation is nonreflective and typically includes three basic features: assuming a comfortable body position, maintaining physical immobility, and continuously focusing attention on some object, sound, or bodily process such as breathing (Kus, 1995). Both are effective in enhancing spirituality and assisting in recovery from alcoholism. The expert panel examining the relationship of spirituality to alcohol and drug problems noted that meditation-based interventions are associated with reduced levels of alcohol/drug use and problems (Larson et al., 1997). Walsh (1999) cautioned that the form of meditation used should fit with each client's spiritual beliefs, preferences, and comfort.

Although meditation may take one of the forms just identified, I suggest a form of meditation in which family members listen to each other and to the "family spirit," even as they listen to their own spirit and perhaps, their higher power. Wright (1999) noted the spiritual benefits that are received when family members coping with serious illness are listened to and it is likely that families coping with alcoholism would benefit similarly. "The inviting, listening to, and witnessing illness stories provides a powerful validation of a profound human experience...Outcomes have been the alleviation of physical symptoms and familial conflict as well as the diminishing or alleviating of emotional and/or spiritual suffering" (Wright, 1999, p. 67). Empathy is a key component of good listening. Encouraging the expression and sharing of feelings in small groups with a facilitator can be particularly helpful in increasing empathy, especially among men (Oliner & Oliner, 1995).

Prayer

Prayer is another activity that facilitates spiritual growth and provides health benefits. Many use prayer to help them cope with a wide range of life's problems and concerns (McCullough & Larson, 1999). Dossey (1993) reviewed numerous medical studies examining the efficacy of prayer in producing physical changes and suggested that the ritual of prayer may trigger emotions that positively impact the cardiovascular and immune systems, leading to changes in health. There is also research that suggests that those who pray may benefit from the activity of prayer. O'Laoire (1997) conducted a study on intercessory prayer (i.e., praying for others) in which agents prayed for randomly-assigned subjects 15 minutes a day for 12 weeks. While all participants, agents as well as subjects, showed improvement on measures of depression, anxiety, and self-esteem, the agents received benefits superior to those received by the subjects. Thus, just praying regularly for family members has the potential to promote spiritual and physical well-being within the family.

Although Americans seem to prefer praying silently and alone (Gallup Organization, 1993), audible prayers for family members in their presence might be especially powerful in terms of healing and nourishing the communal soul. Depending on their comfort level with prayer, family members could be invited at first to assemble and pray silently for one another. In time they could be encouraged to pray audibly for one another. These things could be done in conjunction with meditation or as a separate activity.

An observation by May (1988) bears mentioning here. He noted that persons who are not accustomed to sitting still might have great difficulty with spiritual practices that require spending time in quiet, receptive openness (i.e., meditation and prayer). "The simple matter of taking time for daily prayer can become a battle of will excruciatingly reminiscent of that encountered in chemical addiction" (May, 1988, p. 89). As with any exercise or homework assignment a clinician recommends, clients should be asked about their experiences and the effects of the activities in which they were asked to engage.

Restoring Rituals

Restoring and embellishing the family's ritual life is yet another way to promote healthy family spirituality and strengthen the communal soul. As noted earlier, rituals are severely damaged or lost in many alcoholic families (Steinglass et al., 1987). In addition to restoring meaningful rituals that have been altered or discontinued, families should also be encouraged to create new ones. The new rituals can promote healing by enabling the family to mourn its losses (Imber-Black, 1991), or they can strengthen family connections and enhance the family's communal soul (Imber-Black & Roberts, 1992).

Madanes (1991) described a 16-step reparation ritual she used with families in which sexual abuse had occurred. As part of the ritual, the therapist explains that the sexual abuse caused spiritual pain for both the victim and the victimizer. The therapist then asks the offender to get on his or her knees in front of the victim and sincerely express sorrow and repentance. The therapist next has the other family members get on their knees in front of the victim and express sorrow for having failed to protect the victim. Later steps in the healing process include identifying what can be done as an act of reparation and helping the victimizer to forgive himself or herself.

The ritual just described was designed to heal shame in the family, an important goal in the family therapy model employed by Madanes. Shame and guilt are key issues in the spiritual lives of those with alcohol problems (Kurtz, 1981) and for that reason, the 12 steps of AA encourage alcoholics to acknowledge wrongdoing and take steps to make amends. Given the trauma and shame often experienced in a family as a result of alcoholism, a ritual of the kind used by Madanes might go a long way toward helping the family to let go of its painful past, restore its resources of trust, and look to the future with renewed vision and hope.

Confession and Forgiveness

A regular practice of confession and forgiveness can enable the family to restore and/or improve its spiritual health. Such ethical behaviors promote healthy social interactions and relationships based on honesty, mutual respect, and trust (Hargrave, 1994; Tonigan, Toscova, & Connors, 1999). Furthermore, confession and forgiveness can address and resolve feelings of bitterness that may have developed over time. Bitterness hinders spiritual connection and fulfillment, and frustrates efforts to alter health, stress, or personal relationship patterns (Kurtz & Ketcham, 1992; Martin & Booth, 1999).

The need for confession is obvious when there is a recognized hurt. However, since some offenses are inadvertent and sometimes unrecognized (though no less hurtful), family members might ask one another, "Have I hurt you in any way?" Ferguson, Ferguson, Thurman, Thurman, and Ferguson (1994) outlined a multi-step procedure that family members can use to heal emotional hurts. Family members begin by listing ways in which they have hurt other family members. Then they are encouraged to confess those hurts to God. Next, they each in turn share their lists with the persons they have hurt and request forgiveness for the wrongs they have done, being sure to state that what they did was wrong, rather than simply saying they are sorry. Before moving to the next person, the one confessing hurts is encouraged to ask, "Are there other major hurts that I've not seen that also need my apology?" After all family members have confessed all of the identified hurts, they exchange their lists and tear them up or burn or bury them. Although it is hoped that family members will forgive the confessed wrongs, forgiveness is a choice and there is no obligation to forgive. Family members will sometimes be reluctant to forgive if the depth of sorrow over the wrongs committed does not equal or approximate the depth of the hurt they experienced (Ferguson et al., 1994).

Service to Others

Families recovering from alcoholism might also be encouraged to devote themselves to acts of service. Serving others can be both a means to improve spiritual health and an indicator of spiritual renewal and growth (Anderson, 1999). Many spiritual traditions speak of receiving through giving. Families and family members who give to others and devote themselves to making a difference in their community, receive a host of therapeutic benefits, including increased self-esteem, a renewed sense of meaning in life, a greater vision for the future, and feelings of connectedness (Doherty, 1995; Perry & Rolland, 1999). Of course, there needs to be a balance between self-care and caring for others. Those inclined to be over-responsible and self-sacrificing may first need to learn to value and care for the self. Once that goal is achieved, they can be encouraged to engage again in caring for others.

Religious Involvement

Finally, families might be encouraged to consider becoming involved in a religious community. Religion is a vehicle for many to discover, enhance, or express their spirituality. Those for whom religion is an important influence and a source of comfort are more likely to feel close to their families, find their jobs fulfilling, and be hopeful about the future (Chamberlain & Zika, 1992). For those coping with difficult circumstances, religious practice often brings meaning, solace, and strength, and religious communities can provide friendship and emotional support (Poston & Turnbull, 2004). Gorsuch (1995) reviewed the literature on the relationship between religiousness and substance abuse and concluded that "religiousness involving anti-abuse norms, a loving, supportive, and empowering (rather than restrictive) 'higher authority,' and peers who are anti-substance abuse may all have positive influences on the substance abuser" (p. 78).

As noted earlier, the relationship between religion and spirituality is much debated, with some seeing religious involvement as a hindrance to spiritual growth, rather than a help. Despite the evidence that religious involvement can be beneficial, there is also the potential for harm. Religious experience characterized by non-nurturing control and punishment has been linked to antisocial behavior in general and alcohol abuse in particular (Forliti & Benson, 1986). Therefore, before suggesting religious involvement, it would be important to explore the kind of religion (if any) the family has experienced. Clinicians must guard against suggesting something that is likely to further traumatize persons who have already endured the traumatization of alcoholism (Finnegan & McNally, 1995). The benefits of religious involvement are most often associated with "a caring and supportive religiousness" (Gorsuch, 1995, p. 80). Although clinicians must respect clients' choices with regard to the practice of religion, clients should be assisted in making an informed choice. Some may feel obligated to return to the religion of their childhood, even if that religion was a negativistic, punishing religion. Research has shown that most alcoholics have experienced that kind of religion (Fowler, 1993). If clients automatically return to that religious context, the result might be relapse rather than spiritual growth.

CASE EXAMPLE

Ted M. had received substance abuse treatment for alcoholism in an intensive outpatient treatment program. His aftercare plan included family counseling provided through his employee assistance program. Ted, his wife Beth, and their two sons, ages 12 and 9, attended the initial family session. During the session, Ted disclosed that he had attended a spirituality group during his outpatient treatment and "got a lot out of it." At the same time, he acknowledged that he had not thought much about spirituality since then, except when he attended AA meetings. Beth said that she had grown up in a religious family, but religion and spirituality had played only a very small role in her marriage and family. She said that she had attended church with her two sons when they were young, but as Ted's alcoholism and their other problems grew worse, she gradually gave that up. She also disclosed that she used to pray fairly often, but had quit that as well, because she felt guilty and ashamed. The older son said that he remembered going to church as a child. He said he wondered why they stopped going, but never asked. Beth expressed the hope that her family could become more spiritual again and Ted indicated that he was open to that. Both stated that they would like for that to be part of their family counseling.

In keeping with Ted and Beth's desire, the counselor introduced several spiritually-based practices into the therapy. The first practice was meditation. Ted noted that in his spirituality group, the patients were invited to spend some time in quiet reflection. With their eyes closed, they were to imagine what they wanted their lives to be like, and then imagine their higher power guiding them toward that. The counselor suggested that the family members could do something similar to that, but they could imagine what they wanted their family to be like and then imagine God helping them to achieve that. All family members agreed to try it. Afterwards, they said that it was different, but okay. When meditation was used in the next session, Beth suggested that the family members hold hands as they meditated and all agreed. At the end of the session, the counselor invited them to try doing that at home. Ted suggested that mealtime might be a good time for that.

As counseling progressed, other spiritually-based practices were introduced or recommended. At Beth's request, the family began saying prayers before meals and at bedtime. The bedtime prayers were usually between Beth and each of the boys, but occasionally, Ted also would join them. After several counseling sessions, the counselor asked the family to consider a family service project. Ted stated that a friend had invited him to participate in a "Habitat for Humanity" building project. He proposed that the whole family participate, and the other family members expressed an interest in doing so. At the next session, they reported that they all had a great time together and planned to devote at least one Saturday each month working on a similar project.

Near the end of the family counseling sessions, Beth expressed a desire to attend religious services again. Ted seemed hesitant at first, but then stated that he would be willing to go with her at least a few times. The counselor initiated a discussion about the impact different religious approaches can have on recovery (i.e., a caring and supportive religiousness versus a negativistic, punishing religion). Beth said that she had been thinking about attending a friend's church, but before doing so, she would find out more about it.

At the conclusion of counseling, Ted, Beth, and their sons all agreed that they were a closer, happier family. Although the sessions focused on much more than the family's spirituality, Ted and Beth acknowledged that the spiritually-based practices suggested by the counselor played an important role in the process of change. Of course, not all families will be as open to such practices and, therefore, they may have to be introduced more slowly, if at all. When they can be introduced and encouraged, the family's "communal soul" (Anderson, 1999) can be healed, renewed, and strengthened.

CONCLUSION

There is ample research to show that when spiritual beliefs and practices are included in the treatment of alcoholism, great benefits are possible. The reason for this is clear in the minds of those who advocate spirituality's inclusion. Alcoholism is, at least in part, a spiritual disease with spiritual roots and spiritual implications. In this article, I have attempted to make a case for including spiritual interventions in the treatment of families whose communal soul has been damaged due to alcoholism.

Spirituality is a controversial subject, evoking a great deal of emotion, both positive and negative. While some embrace and support the notion that human beings are spiritual by nature, others strongly deny and reject that proposition. Some families will not embrace their spirituality or the spiritual practices that have the potential to enhance their spiritual life and growth. With such families, spirituality issues must be introduced into treatment very carefully. For families who are open, or become open, to spiritual conversations and spiritual interventions, there can be tremendous benefits.

Kurtz and Ketcham (1992) used the metaphor of architecture in talking about addressing spirituality with clients. What are required, they said, are tools, a plan, and a commitment to do the work. I have identified several tools that can be used to encourage clients' spiritual growth. It is the clinician's responsibility to work with families to develop a plan and commit themselves to it.

REFERENCES

Alcoholics Anonymous. (1976). *Alcoholics Anonymous* (3rd ed.). New York: Alcoholics Anonymous World Services, Inc.

Anderson, H. (1999). Feet planted firmly in midair: A spirituality for family living. In F. Walsh (Ed.), *Spiritual resources in family therapy* (pp. 157-176). New York: Guilford.

Aponte, H. J. (1999). The stresses of poverty and the comfort of spirituality. In F. Walsh (Ed.), *Spiritual resources in family therapy* (pp. 157-176). New York: Guilford.

Beavers, W. R., & Hampson, R. B. (1990). *Successful families: Assessment and intervention.* New York: Norton.

Brawer, P. A., Handal, P. J., Fabricatore, A. N., Roberts, R., & Wajda-Johnston, V. A. (2002). Training and education in religion/spirituality within APA-accredited clinical psychology programs. *Professional Psychology: Research and Practice, 33,* 203-206.

Carlson, T. D., & Erickson, M. J. (2000). Re-authoring spiritual narratives: God in persons' relational identity stories. *Journal of Systemic Therapies, 19,* 65-83.

Chamberlain, K., & Zika, S. (1992). Religiosity, meaning in life, and psychological well-being. In J. Schumaker (Ed.), *Religion and mental health* (pp. 138-148). New York: Oxford University Press.

Doherty, W. (1995). *Soul searching: Why psychotherapy must promote moral responsibility.* New York: Basic Books.

Dossey, L. (1993). *Healing words.* New York: HarperCollins.

Edwards, M. E., & Steinglass, P. (1995). Family therapy treatment outcomes for alcoholism. *Journal of Marital and Family Therapy, 21,* 475-509.

Ferguson, D., Ferguson, T., Thurman, C., Thurman, H., & Ferguson, T. (1994). *Intimate encounters: A practical guide to discovering the secrets of a really great marriage.* Nashville, TN: Thomas Nelson.

Finnegan, D. G., & McNally, E. B. (1995). Defining God or a Higher Power: The spiritual center of recovery. In R. Kus (Ed.), *Spirituality and chemical dependency* (pp. 39-48). New York: Haworth.

Forliti, J. E., & Benson, P. L. (1986). Young adolescents: A national study. *Religious Education, 8,* 199-224.

Fowler, J. W. (1993). Alcoholics Anonymous and faith development. In B. S. McCrady & W. R. Miller (Eds.), *Research on Alcoholics Anonymous: Opportunities and alternatives* (pp. 113-135). New Brunswick, NJ: Rutgers Center of Alcohol Studies.

Fukuyama, M. A., & Sevig, T. D. (1997). Spiritual issues in counseling: A new course. *Therapist Education and Supervision, 36,* 233-244.

Gallup Organization. (1993). *GO LIFE Survey on Prayer.* Princeton, NJ: Author.

Gorsuch, R. L. (1993). Assessing spiritual variables in Alcoholics Anonymous research. In B. S. McCrady & W. R. Miller (Eds.), *Research on Alcoholics Anonymous: Opportunities and alternatives.* New Brunswick, NJ: Rutgers Center of Alcohol Studies.

Gorsuch, R. L. (1995). Religious aspects of substance abuse and recovery. *Journal of Social Issues, 51,* 65-83.

Hargrave, T. D. (1994). *Families & forgiveness: Healing wounds in the intergenerational family.* New York: Brunner/Mazel.

Imber-Black, E. (1991). Rituals and the healing process. In F. Walsh & M. McGoldrick (Eds.), *Living beyond loss: Death in the family* (pp. 207-223). New York: W.W. Norton.

Imber-Black, E., & Roberts, J. (1992). *Rituals for our times: Celebrating, healing, and changing our lives and our relationships.* New York: HarperCollins.

Kurtz, E. (1979). *Not-God: A history of Alcoholics Anonymous.* Minneapolis, MN: Hazelden.

Kurtz, E. (1981). *Shame and guilt: Characteristics of the dependency cycle.* Minneapolis, MN: Hazelden.

Kurtz, E., & Ketcham, K. (1992). *The spirituality of imperfection: Storytelling and the journey to wholeness.* New York: Bantam Books.

Kus, R. J. (1995). Prayer and meditation in addiction recovery. In R. Kus (Ed.), *Spirituality and chemical dependency* (pp. 39-48). New York: Haworth.

Larson, D. B., Swyers, J. P., & McCullough, M. E. (Eds.). (1997). *Scientific research on spirituality and health: A consensus report.* Rockville, MD: National Institute for Healthcare Research.

Madanes, C. (1991). Strategic family therapy. In A. S. Gurman & D. P. Kniskern (Eds.), *Handbook of Family Therapy (Vol. II)* (pp. 396-416). New York: Brunner/Mazel.

Martin, J. E., & Booth, J. (1999). Behavioral approaches to enhance spirituality. In W. R. Miller (Ed.), *Integrating spirituality into treatment: Resources for practitioners* (pp. 161-175). Washington, DC: American Psychological Association.

Martin, J. E., & Carlson, C. R. (1988). Spiritual dimensions of health psychology. In W. R. Miller & J. E. Martin (Eds.), *Behavior therapy and religion: Integrating spiritual and behavioral approaches to change* (pp. 57-110). Newbury Park, CA: Sage.

May, G. G. (1988). *Addiction & grace: Love and spirituality in the healing of addictions.* San Francisco, CA: HarperCollins.

May, G. G. (1991). *The awakened heart: Opening yourself to the love you need.* San Francisco, CA: HarperCollins.

McCullough, M. E., & Larson, D. B. (1999). Prayer. In W. R. Miller (Ed.), *Integrating spirituality into treatment: Resources for practitioners* (pp. 85-110). Washington, DC: American Psychological Association.

Miller, W. R. (1990). Spirituality: The silent dimension in addiction research. *Drug and Alcohol Review, 9,* 259-266.

Miller, W. R. (1999). Diversity training in spiritual and religious issues. In W. R. Miller (Ed.), *Integrating spirituality into treatment: Resources for practitioners* (pp. 253-263). Washington, DC: American Psychological Association.

Miller, W. R., & Thoresen, C. E. (1999). Spirituality and health. In W. R. Miller (Ed.), *Integrating spirituality into treatment: Resources for practitioners* (pp. 3-18). Washington, DC: American Psychological Association.

O'Laoire, S. (1997). An experimental study of the effects of distant, intercessory prayer on self-esteem, anxiety, and depression. *Alternative Therapies in Health and Medicine, 3,* 38-53.

Oliner, P. M., & Oliner, S. P. (1995). *Toward a caring society.* Westport, CT: Praeger.

Ornish, D., Brown, S. E., Scherwitz, L. W., Billings, J. H., Armstrong, W. T., & Ports, T. A. (1990). Can coronary artery disease be reversed? *Lancet, 336,* 129-133.

Peck, M. S. (1993). *Further along the road less traveled: The unending journey toward spiritual growth.* New York: Simon & Schuster.

Perry, A. D. V., & Rolland, J. S. (1999). Spirituality expressed in community action: A therapeutic means to liberation and hope. In F. Walsh (Ed.), *Spiritual resources in family therapy* (pp. 272-292). New York: Guilford.

Poston, D. J., & Turnbull, A. P. (2004). Role of spirituality and religion in family quality of life for families of children with disabilities. *Education and Training in Developmental Disabilities, 39*, 95-108.

Royce, J. E. (1995). The effects of alcoholism and recovery on spirituality. In R. Kus (Ed.), *Spirituality and chemical dependency* (pp. 19-37). New York: Haworth.

Samford, B., Vaughn, M., Shumway, S., Jefferies, V., & Arredondo, R. (2001). Treating individuals and families for alcohol/other drug problems in an intensive outpatient setting. *Alcoholism Treatment Quarterly, 19*, 65-80.

Steinglass, P., Bennett, L. A., Wolin, S. J., & Reiss, D. (1987). *The alcoholic family.* New York: BasicBooks.

Steinglass, P., Tislenko, L., & Reiss, D. (1985). Stability/instability in the alcoholic marriage: The interrelationships between course of alcoholism, family process, and marital outcome. *Family Process, 24*, 365-376.

Stinnett, N., & DeFrain, J. (1985). *Secrets of strong families.* Boston: Little, Brown.

Tonigan, J. S., Toscova, R. T., & Connors, G. J. (1999). Spirituality and the 12-step programs: A guide for clinicians. In W. R. Miller (Ed.), *Integrating spirituality into treatment: Resources for practitioners* (pp. 111-131). Washington, DC: American Psychological Association.

Walsh, F. (1999). Religion and spirituality. In F. Walsh (Ed.), *Spiritual resources in family therapy* (pp. 3-27). New York: Guilford.

Wright, L. M. (1999). Spirituality, suffering, and beliefs. In F. Walsh (Ed.), *Spiritual resources in family therapy* (pp. 61-75). New York: Guilford.

doi:10.1300/J020v25n01_09

Index